Walking Through Pregnancy and Beyond

HOW EXPECTANT AND NEW MOMS CAN WALK THEIR WAY THROUGH A HAPPY AND HEALTHY PREGNANCY AND FIRST YEAR

By Mark and Lisa Fenton   With Tracy Teare

THE LYONS PRESS
Guilford, Connecticut

An imprint of The Globe Pequot Press

The following provided photographs for the book: Vito Aluia: 16; Baby Bjorn: 108, 113; Baby Jogger:192; Bob Strollers: 111, 147, 150; Judith Broggi: 156, 157; Burley: 144, 202, 204, 207 (top), 214; Mark Fenton: 43, 101, 115, 136, 194, 195, 197, 201, 207 (bottom); Evan Cece Garner: 7; Ann Halbower: 77, 154; Gary Higgins: xiii, 2, 12, 19, 24, 26, 27, 28, 29, 46, 47, 54, 56, 58, 63, 66, 67, 78, 79, 83, 84, 90, 138, 149, 168, 170, 171; Keller & Keller: 181, 182, 183; Michael Lanza: 41, 52, 164 (top), 172, 176, 178, 188, 191; John Librett: 55; Elizabeth McGuire: 48; Mothers in Motion: 9, 15, 80, 82, 128; Sue Ryder: 75; Tracy Teare: 104, 110; Samantha Weld: 99.

The Lyons Press is an imprint of The Globe Pequot Press

10 9 8 7 6 5 4 3 2 1

Printed in the United States of America

Designed by LeAnna Weller Smith

ISBN 1-59228-384-5

Library of Congress Cataloging-in-Publication Data is available on file

For Maxwell and Skye, Caitlin, Ellie, and Natalie.
Thanks for teaching us all we need to learn.

cont

ents

Acknowledgments

Many researchers and clinicians contributed to the extensive literature we reviewed for this book, and it would be impossible to thank them all. However, we would like to acknowledge those professionals who gave their time for interviews, or who helped clear up specific issues or technical questions. Special thanks to:

Raul Artal, MD, professor and chairman of the Department of Obstetrics, Gynecology, and Women's Health at the St. Louis University School of Medicine; William Boyle, MD, a pediatrician at the Children's Hospital at Dartmouth in Lebanon, New Hampshire, and a fellow of the American Academy of Pediatrics; Colette Crawford, RN, BSN, master yoga instructor and founder of the Seattle Holistic Center; Danielle Symons Downs, PhD, assistant professor of kinesiology, Pennsylvania State University; Andrea Dunn, PhD, at the Cooper Institute for Aerobics Research, in Denver; Ann Halbower, MD, medical director of the Pediatric Sleep Disorders Program at Johns Hopkins University School of Medicine; Ann Hansen, MD, a neonatologist at the Children's Hospital in Boston; Melvin B. Heyman, MD, MPH, professor of pediatrics and chief of pediatric gastroenterology, hepatology, and nutrition at the University of California, San Francisco; Kirsten Krahnstoever Davison, PhD, at Pennsylvania State University; Michelle Mottola, PhD, director of the R. Samuel McLaughlin Foundation Exercise and Pregnancy Laboratory at the University of Western Ontario; Marjorie C. Meyer, MD, associate professor of obstetrics and gynecology, University of Vermont School of Medicine; Robert Pangrazi, PhD, a professor at Arizona State University; JoAnn Rohyans, MD, a spokesperson for the American Academy of Pediatrics and member of the Pediatric Department at the Ohio State University College of Medicine; Elizabeth Ward, MS, RD, a nutritionist and author based in Boston.

Thanks to the manufacturers who helped us understand the world of baby hardware, and shared many fine photo images sprinkled through the book, including Ann Obenchine (Kelty®), Elisabeth Bergoo (Baby Björn®), Damon Noller (Bob Strollers™), John Kluge and Ronnel Curry (Burley®), and Teri Durrin (Dreamer Design). Special thanks to Ed and Bess Hilpert at Mothers in Motion maternity wear for their extra help with photography.

Most of all, we appreciate the many mothers who indulged our extensive and probing curiosity and who shared their stories and insights. They're the real experts, and we're all lucky to be able to learn from their experiences. Special thanks to Pam Ahl, Ginny Ayers, Penny Beach, Pat Brennan, Susan Campbell, Kathy Detwiler, Colleen Ellis, Joy Fawcett, Evan Cece Garner, Diana Grenier, Dana Kilroy, Wendy King, Allison Librett, Elizabeth McGuire, Melinda Miller, Lisa Rafferty, Cathy Robinson, Lindsay Rosenthal, Cindy Ross, Sue Ryder, Cara Seiderman, Wendy Sharp, Kim Sutton, Peg Treadwell, Larah Walker, Samantha Weld, Lochen Wood, and many others with whom we chatted informally along the way. Also thanks to Kevin Weafer, our dear friend and former publisher of *Walking* magazine, and still dedicated walking advocate.

Most important, thanks to our parents for encouraging and enabling our active lifestyles starting from the very beginning.

Final thanks to four people critical to the completion of this work. Photographer Gary Higgins was a professional and personal joy. Pregnant mom Cindia Nelson is not just a wonderful photo model, but role model as well. Designer LeAnna Weller Smith graciously persevered against all of our disorganizational odds to miraculously pull the design together. And Editor Ann Treistmen showed persistent faith in ably and patiently negotiating the trickiest of waters—coordinating the work of a husband and wife writing team!

Thanks so much for helping to make this idea a reality.

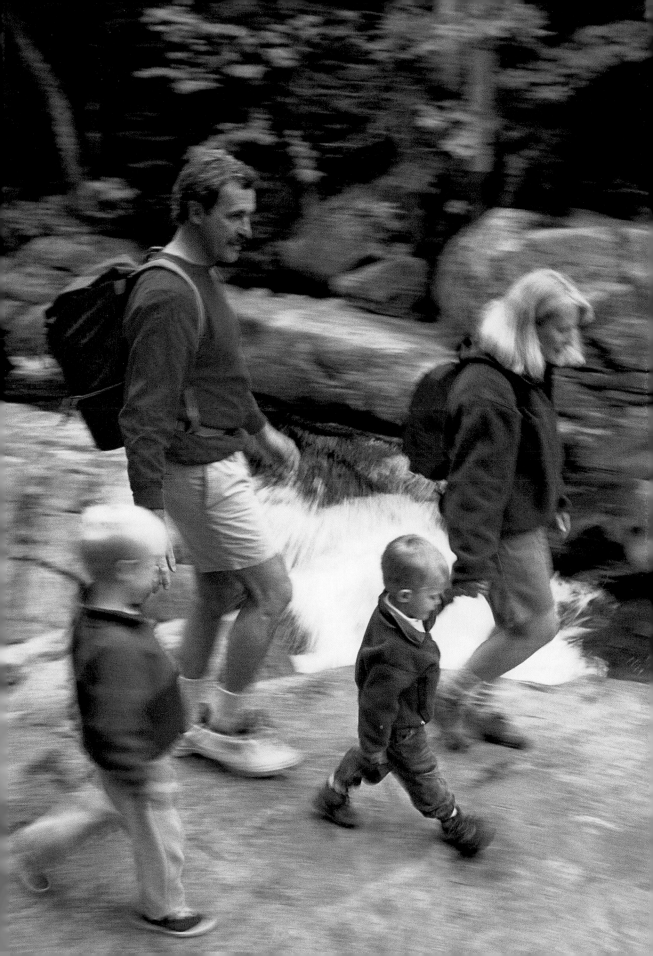

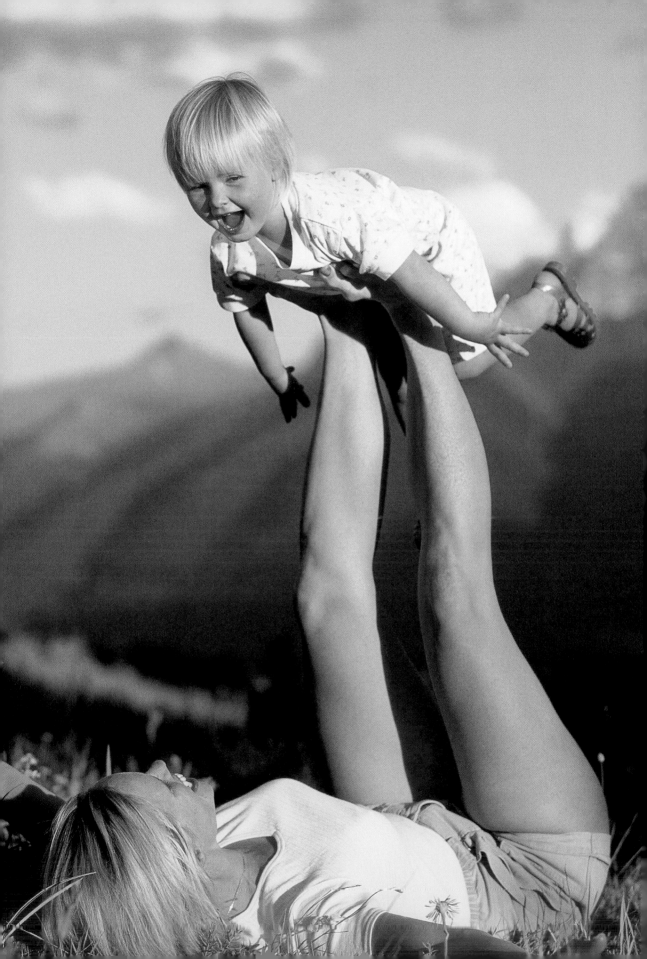

Introduction

This book has a very simple pattern. That means you should be able to read it either straight through, like a novel—say, *The Amazing Story of You, Your Baby, and Walking*—or more like a reference manual, if you prefer. It's broken into seven sections, which roughly reflect seven phases most women go through from the beginning of pregnancy ("I'm *what?*") to a year after the baby is born. ("A shower, I need a shower. And some sleep.") Each is either a trimester of three months before delivery, or a postmester (yeah, it's a made-up word, but we like it) of three months afterward.

Each section has the same pattern: An opening chapter summarizes the science, sprinkled with stories of women's experiences to illustrate that we are not making this stuff up. Then there's a brief chapter on gear that might be useful at this stage in the game. And finally comes the program chapter—variously detailed instructions on appropriate exercises that will help keep you fit, and healthy, and comfortable, and most of all happy, plus a recommended walking program for the three-month period in question.

Two important things about that third chapter, the exercise program. It's not really that specific. It gives a broad outline and suggested routine of walking and complementary exercises for several different levels of effort and fitness. But it's intentionally broad and lacking in rigidity because of what's going on in your life, by definition, if you're reading this book. So don't be looking for "Monday—45 minutes at 75 percent of maximum heart rate," because we're not going to give it to you. What we'll say instead is, *At this stage of your pregnancy, if everything's going well and you feel all right and the doctor is okay with it, then a typical week of exercise should look like this.* You decide exactly which days to do what, and exactly what intensity—make it fit your schedule, your lifestyle, how you feel.

But none of that flexibility is designed to let you off the hook. You need to get moving, and we mean now. And walking is the best possible choice.

Another thing. This book looks like a standard exercise book, and in many ways it is— stretches, warm-ups, program recommendations . . . But it's based on a slightly different premise than much of the exercise pabulum that's out there. The difference is our fundamental philosophy: If you try to carve special time out of your life exclusively for exercise and you depend on that, you're eventually doomed to failure. Sure, it may work for a while—even the 21 months represented by this book. Traditional approaches like taking a class or going to the gym might even be enough to keep you fit through pregnancy, and help you lose any

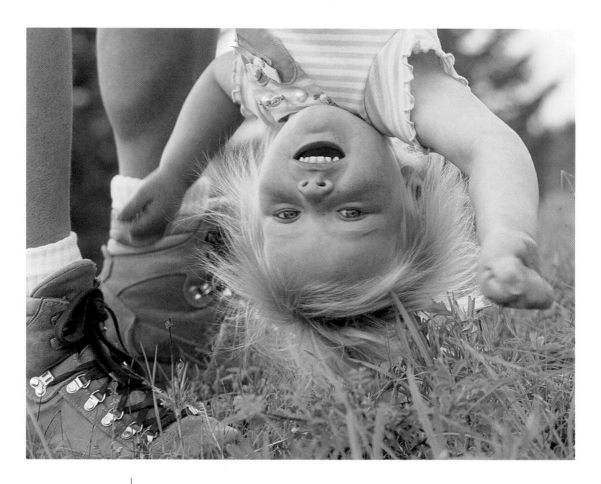

excess weight successfully afterward. But in the long run, it has flaws. First, it's very susceptible to life changes—you move away from the gym, or your favorite instructor does, or they boost their fees, or you get a new job, or have another child—and it can fall apart. Second, it's always competing for time with all the other things you have to do—going to work and the store, taking care of the house, and, most costly, being with your new child. That's where our philosophy comes in.

We believe that the core—the absolute centerpiece—of your exercise should be creating an active lifestyle around walking. Take an exercise class, go to the gym, do it all. But make the heart of your activity walking every day. It's ultimately flexible. You can walk anytime, anyplace, it costs you nothing, there's no instructor needed (this book will give you all you need)—and walking is always with you, wherever life takes you. Best of all, you can and should build walking into other things you do—walk for shopping and errands, walk to the bus and to work, walk your older child(ren) to school and to soccer practice and a friend's house. Walk your dog, walk to relieve stress, walk just to be outside.

We also believe you have to share this lifestyle with your baby. It's not just a good idea, it's an absolute obligation. America is suffering obesity epidemics among both its adult and its youth populations, and 30 minutes of walking (the surgeon general's recommendation for daily physical activity) would go a long way toward stemming the tide of what Dr. Julie Geberding, head of the Centers for Disease Control, has called America's number one health problem. Here's the scary thing: How much we walk–or, more to the point, *don't* walk–really matters. There's growing evidence that a lifestyle of driving everywhere, spending increasing time in front of computer and TV screens, eating less at home and more out, and living in communities where it's harder and harder to walk to school or the corner store is a tremendous contributor to the rising tide of obesity. Forty years ago, two-thirds or more of children walked to school; now fewer than 15 percent do. That leads to the final part of our philosophy.

If you really care about your children's long-term welfare, you have to be an agent of change. You can start by simply walking in your community and being a role model. Get out on foot, with your child, and remind people that yes, it can be done. But don't stop there. As you walk, you'll see what works. Things like compact communities with sidewalks and corner stores and traditional walkable downtowns; neighborhood elementary schools and parks and playgrounds; old rail corridors with biking and walking trails. And you'll see what doesn't: sprawl-

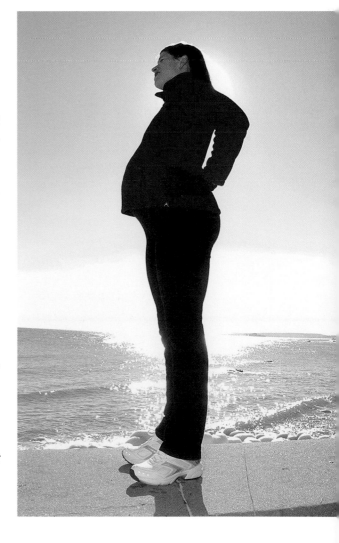

ing suburbs with wide, fast roads and no sidewalks; giant centralized school districts where every student is bussed 30 minutes each way; strip malls and big-box stores and impassable high-speed, six-lane roads. And once you've learned to recognize it, you'll want to do something about it. Start a walk-to-school program, get sidewalks built, if necessary move to a safer community. You're bringing another life into this world, and it shouldn't be a life that's doomed to sedentary living, obesity, and an elevated risk for a host of chronic diseases.

It should be a life that learns how to cross streets safely and be healthy and be observant and walk with friends. And a life that learns the shortcut to a friend's house over the creek, and knows what it is to walk on a warm summer night and see fireflies, or on a cold winter day when your breath freezes on your eyebrows. It should be a life so used to being physically active that walking is just an intrinsic part of existence. And only you can make this introduction, and help create that more walkable world.

We hope this book will help you walk through pregnancy. We hope it will help you walk with your child, after he or she arrives. And we hope it will help you walk beyond, way beyond, to the point that you're helping others come along with you.

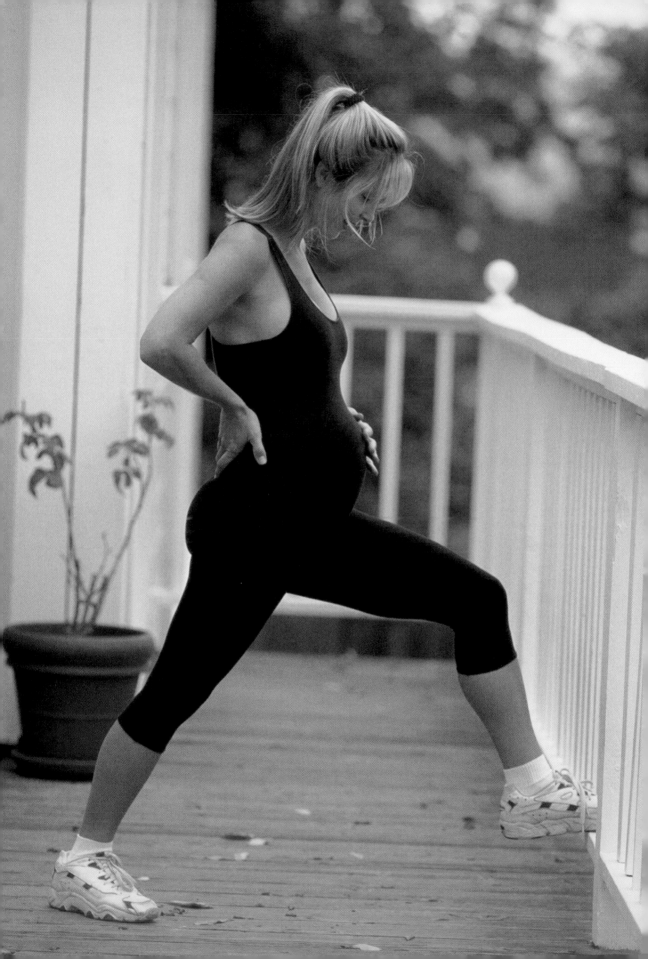

Staying Active While Building a Baby

The Answer in a Nutshell

Congratulations: You're about to experience one of the most exciting adventures of your life. But rather than go on about life's greatest miracle, and the extraordinary joy and challenge you're about to face—you can get that from lots of other books—we're going to come right out and give you the single gem for which you're reading this book. You're looking for advice, you want to know how to do it right for both your baby and yourself, and we can boil our pearl of wisdom down to two words: *Keep moving.* One word, actually: *Walk!* That's it, that's what you got this book for, so there it is: Walk.

"But wait," you might say, "I'm a first-time mother and I don't know about pregnancy and I'm a little nervous and want to do everything absolutely right." Okay, here's our advice: Walk. Every day.

"But I'm really no super athlete—I don't have much of an exercise habit at all." Fine. Walk a little less, build it up very gradually. But walk.

"No, you don't understand," you might object. "I'm overweight, and really concerned about my ankles and knees and hips, plus the weight I'm going to gain with the baby . . ." All the more reason, we say, to walk. Start slow and easy. Stop if anything starts to hurt (trust us, it won't—walking is low impact and joint-friendly). But walk. Starting right now.

"But won't exercise give me a low-weight baby? Don't I risk early labor? Can't I hurt myself for future pregnancies by exercising now?" The simple answers are no, no, and no. In fact, walking is the favorite recommendation of the medical profession, the benefits are so great and the risks so low.

"Sure, but I'm a serious runner and aerobics instructor. Are you going to tell me *walking* is going to keep me fit through this pregnancy?" Yes! Walking can be as hard-core and challenging as you want (we'll prove it) and with vastly less risk than higher-impact activities.

"Hey, I've got older kids, and a job, and a house to take care of, and lots of responsibilities. How will I have time?" Listen closely, because this may be the most important part of our gem. You can take the older kids along—that's why they make strollers, and bikes, and scooters. You can walk over lunch hour. You can throw in the laundry 20 minutes later. But right now, walk. The greatest responsibility you have for the next nine months and beyond is to the health and welfare of your baby and you. And one of the best things you can do for both of you is—surprise—walk!

Walk every day and you'll remain healthier and more fit. You'll gain less excess weight during the pregnancy, and be more likely to get walking (and lose that weight) after the delivery. You'll deal with nausea and sleepless nights and raging hormones better, and simply feel better about yourself through it all. You'll go into the delivery more fit and prepared, and come out more ready to deal with a new baby in your life. Keep it up after delivery, and you'll begin establishing a healthy habit for *two* lifetimes—yours and your child's. You'll lose the extra weight. You'll be less stressed out. You'll simply feel better.

Now you're thinking, *These folks are fanatics and they think walking is the silver bullet. The great preventive and cure-all elixir. A magical potion that helps you live a longer and healthier life, and have a better pregnancy to boot.*

Don't be silly. There's no such thing. But here's the kicker—a daily walk is absolutely, positively as close as you can get. It is humankind's best medicine. And there's plenty of research to back up this heady assertion. So whether you call it an early-morning stroll, an after-dinner constitutional, a daily power walk, a rambling chat with your sister, a 15-minute amble to the bus and 15 minutes back, a walk with the dog, a hike in the hills, or 30 minutes away from the telephone, a walk is what you need. Every day. From now until your bundle of joy arrives, and then every day after that, with the joy-bundle along for the ride.

First, talk to your doctor, to make sure you don't have any of the (quite rare) confounding circumstances that make walking a bad idea. Then read on and figure out how much walking is likely right for you—though how you feel is a pretty good guide there. We'll start off with a quiz that will provide a little insight. We'll throw in some ideas and simple exercises to complement your walking. We'll provide

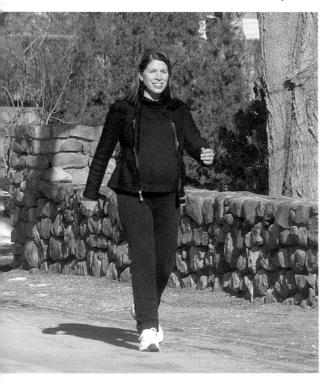

motivational tips from real women who've been through it all, gear that will make it easier along the way, and answers to your most common questions. So read, get comfortable with the science, and get familiar with our "program." And then get out and—you guessed it—take a walk.

BUT HOW MUCH TO WALK?

Don't worry, we'll offer advice that's as specific as you want it to be. This book is divided into sections, each representing three months of your life. That's three trimesters of pregnancy, and four "postmesters" after the baby's born, to guide your exercise all the way through your child's first birthday. Three exercise programs (*low-key, moderate,* and *challenging*) are outlined at the end of this section ("Trimester I") and after each succeeding section of the book. They include general physical activity guidelines and walking recommendations, suggested warm-up, stretching, and strength moves, and a specific sample week that puts it all together if you want that level of detail. There's even a quiz at the beginning of the program to help you determine which level is right for you. But before those details, first let us help you understand why walking is so important to a healthy, happy pregnancy.

Research Rundown: Benefits of a Fit Pregnancy

Gone are the days when pregnant women were told to put their feet up on a couch and take it easy. Instead of the once pervasive fear that activity might harm baby, researchers are continually finding more evidence that exercise is good for pregnant women and their babies.

The number of benefits may even rival the length of your Babies "R" Us shopping list. First, consider the pluses for baby. Exercise has been shown to boost placental growth and result in leaner babies. Even strenuous activity—think competitive athletes—is okay in most cases, and has not been consistently linked with harming baby's health or growth. "There is some conflicting information, but if a pregnant woman eats well and compensates for the calorie loss from exercise, the baby's weight shouldn't be affected by exercise," says Raul Artal, MD, professor and chairman of the Department of Obstetrics, Gynecology, and Women's Health at the St. Louis University School of Medicine. Finally, aerobic exercise, which gets your heart and lungs pumping harder, improves circulation so your body can deliver oxygen to baby more efficiently.

Mothers-to-be get all the regular bonuses of exercise and then some. Staying active keeps off excess weight, helps prevent gestational diabetes, and gives you a head start for getting in shape after baby arrives. Studies have also shown that fit women have an advantage in delivery and recovery. "Fit women don't have shorter or easier labors, but they may have a better tolerance of pain, and they recover much more easily," says Artal. Women who stay fit are also more likely to resume aerobic activities before six weeks postpartum. And those who are active before pregnancy seem less likely to develop a split in the abdominal muscles, which may happen during the third trimester or after delivery.

More good news: Exercise helps pregnant women in countless ways that you won't need to wait nine months to appreciate. Staying active has been shown to help women take in stride the way their changing bodies look. And at a time when hormonal fluctuations may have you reeling, being active can improve your mood, as well as help you cope with stress and boost energy levels. It also eases the myriad side effects that come with pregnancy: constipation, leg cramps, varicose veins, hemorrhoids, poor posture, backaches, and troubled sleep.

What's Happening Inside

Even just a few weeks into your pregnancy, it's probably clear that your body is not its usual self. Maybe you're seeing much more of the bathroom, either because suddenly you need to urinate every other minute or you've won the morning

Nine Ways Exercise Benefits Pregnant Women

1. Prevents excess weight gain.
2. Gives you a head start in regaining pre-pregnancy shape after delivery.
3. Prevents pregnancy-related illness, such as gestational diabetes.
4. Helps you cope with labor, and recover more quickly afterward.
5. Boosts mood and energy levels.
6. Helps you handle stress.
7. Minimizes some of pregnancy's unpleasant side effects.
8. Helps you accept your new body shape more readily.
9. Increases the likelihood you'll return to exercise sooner after delivery.

Staying Active Even with Nausea

About eight weeks into her pregnancy, Lindsay Rosenthal, right, began experiencing what every pregnant woman dreads: full-blown nausea and vomiting. At its height it lasted 24/7 for a month, at which point she went to her doctor, who prescribed medication. At six months pregnant, she still felt queasy on and off.

On the other hand, Evan Cece Garner, at two months pregnant, hadn't vomited, but felt on the verge of it almost every waking moment.

Because the promise that this miserable side effect typically fades away at the end of the first trimester may not be particularly helpful right now, Lindsay and Evan offer these tips on how to cope.

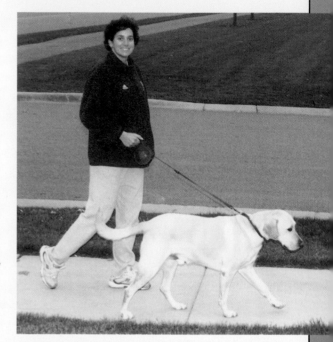

■ Try moving. Even at her worst, Lindsay felt it was better to walk than to sit and suffer: "I'd stop, drink some water, and keep going. Getting out and getting fresh air made me feel better. It was better to get out and move, even if I was sick." For Evan, walking and swimming brought full relief that sometimes lasted half an hour after exercise.

■ Carry cold water and drink plenty of it. Lindsay toted an insulated water bottle filled with ice cubes and water on each outing. "The ice cubes still melt eventually, but the insulation helps shield the water from all the heat in my hands."

■ Eat regularly and avoid an empty stomach. Eat something substantial right after exercising to keep your stomach calmer. Evan's favorites: peanut butter sandwiches and bananas.

■ Avoid positions and modify postures that might make nausea worse, such as forward bends in yoga.

■ "People recommend ginger, licorice, seasickness bands, acupressure. The only thing that's worked for me is mind over matter," says Evan. "Lying down makes me just as nauseous as standing, and since walking is great for the circulatory system, I try to focus on that. This is the most important job I will ever have, and that motivates me beyond anything."

■ Remember that rest is healthy, too. Strive for a balance.

sickness lottery. Add tender, enlarged breasts, strange food cravings, fatigue, and constipation to the list of possible changes you're now experiencing, and you're getting the message loud and clear that you're in for more than a few radical transformations in the upcoming months.

With baby growing inside, the most obvious change will of course be your body shape and weight. In the first trimester, women typically gain 3 to 5 pounds, and then about a pound a week from then on. That should add up to 25 to 35 pounds for the entire pregnancy—less if you're overweight; more if you're underweight or carrying more than one baby. While it's hard to ignore the outward effects of pregnancy, amazing things are happening behind the scenes. In the first three months, the placenta develops, and the major organs and nervous system form. The heart starts to beat, the lungs start to develop, and that tiny head—even face, toes, and fingers—start to form. At the end of this trimester, baby is about the length of your thumb.

HOW EXERCISE AFFECTS BABY

You're probably familiar with at least a simplified version of how your body responds when you get into action. Jump on the treadmill or stride off for a walk, and your heart responds by working harder to move blood to your muscles. Your cardiovascular system kicks into high gear to keep up with the effort, and you start to heat up. But how does this gearing up of your systems affect baby?

Exercise has four major effects on the baby inside you. In normal, low-risk pregnancies, there are protective mechanisms in place that prevent each of these effects from potentially causing harm to the baby. Let's look at these one by one. First, because your body is calling up blood to its muscles to help you move, there is a decrease in the blood flow to the uterus. To counteract this, a built-in mechanism favors the placenta, so that even as blood flow is reduced, the placenta gets priority. Second, this reduction in blood flow to the uterus may mean that less oxygen is delivered

How Big Is Baby, Trimester I?

By the end of the first trimester, the fetus is about 2.5 inches long.

Key developments: Placenta develops, major organs and systems form, tiny human features such as face, toes, and fingers appear.

What this means for you: All this critical development can throw your body for a loop. Be prepared for fatigue, mood fluctuations, maybe nausea and vomiting. And expect to ratchet down your walking program accordingly.

to baby. Again, the placenta compensates with a special response mechanism that helps facilitate the transfer of oxygen and enables baby to use that oxygen more efficiently. Third, when you exercise, your body draws carbohydrates for energy. Though these carbs were potential nourishment for baby, again, the smart placenta reacts by providing alternative food sources. As long as you're eating the recommended nutritious diet for pregnant women and compensate for any calories that you burn off during exercise, this isn't an issue. Fourth and finally, exercise elevates your body's temperature. In this case, Mom's system provides the safety net. Your body adapts by sending more blood flow toward the skin, where the extra heat can dissipate and eliminate potential harm to baby.

Provided you have a normal, uncomplicated pregnancy and follow the recommendations for mild to moderate exercise, these mechanisms counter any potential risks to baby. "We don't know exactly where the threshold is where problems develop, but we do know that with a low-risk pregnancy, these mechanisms are in place for mild to moderate exercise," explains Michelle Mottola, PhD, director of the R. Samuel McLaughlin Foundation Exercise and Pregnancy Lab at the University of Western Ontario. "That's why you err on the side of caution, especially in the first trimester when baby is developing and most susceptible to any of these potential risks. This isn't the time for competing or running marathons."

KEY GUIDELINES FOR FIRST-TRIMESTER EXERCISE

- If your pregnancy is complicated or high risk, your doctor may partially or completely restrict physical activity.

- If you weren't exercising before you got pregnant, check with your doctor before you start. He or she may advise you to wait until the second trimester to begin a progressive exercise program, but a simple walking schedule is probably fine.

- If you were active before pregnancy, it's okay to stay active in the first trimester, but wait until the second trimester to increase the duration, intensity, or frequency of aerobic exercise. Not only are the risks to baby minimal then, but fatigue and nausea should no longer be limiting factors for you.

Why Walking Is Perfect for Pregnancy

Benefits aside, it's essential that pregnant women keep an eye toward safety when they choose sports and activities. When you consider the precautions for exercise during pregnancy, it's easy to see why walking is an ideal choice.

- **WALKING IS THE PHYSICIAN'S FAVORITE.** You're more likely to get the green light from your doctor to walk, even if you weren't exercising before you became pregnant. For normal pregnancies without complications, there's no reason why you can't—and many reasons why you should—get regular moderate exercise, such as walking. If you haven't been exercising, it's important to check with your doctor first. (The same goes if your pregnancy is anything *but* routine. If you have preeclampsia, incompetent cervix, or a history of miscarriage or high blood pressure, for example, you need special guidance, or your doc may restrict activity.)

- **WALKING IS ON THE "SAFE" LIST.** Unlike skiing, horseback riding, bicycling, and in-line skating, walking won't put you or your baby at risk for injury due to a fall (particularly as your balance gets affected by your growing belly). Certainly there's no risk of decompression sickness for baby, such as with scuba diving (also a no-no for pregnant women). And unlike soccer, hockey, and racquetball, there's little chance you'll suffer a potentially damaging collision while you're out for a walk. Still, even the most graceful need to remember that as your belly grows, your center of gravity will shift, compromising your balance, and making you more unsteady as your pregnancy progresses. A safety tip for hikers: As pregnancy progresses, stick to gentle terrain and reliable trails, and altitudes of less than 6,000 feet. Thin air at higher altitudes makes it harder for you and baby to get the oxygen you need.

- **WALKING IS LOW IMPACT.** When you walk, even fast, you only strike the ground with a force equal to one to one-and-a-half times your body weight. Running, by comparison, generates shocks that are three to four times body weight. When you're pregnant, hormones cause the ligaments that support your joints to loosen up, making you more susceptible to injury. That's why nonjarring, nonbouncing, nonpounding activities—like walking and swimming—are so fitting now.

- **WALKING IS ADAPTABLE.** Whether you've been running 10Ks or you're starting an exercise program for the first time, there's a walking program that matches your fitness level and the needs of your particular pregnancy. A walking workout is easily adjusted to maintain a safe heart rate and avoid overheating. Plus, it's easy to downshift when you need to—for instance, if you're experiencing lots of nausea in the first trimester, or when your body is carrying the most weight and tires more easily in the third.

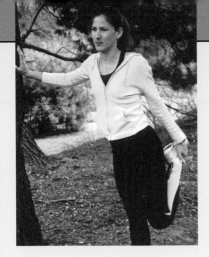

Walking Is a Workout for Everyone

Evan Cece Garner, 39, Austin, Texas.

Even a marathon coach can find walking satisfying during pregnancy. Just ask Evan, above. She's also a duathlete, personal trainer, massage therapist, and anatomy and physiology instructor—and when we spoke with her she was two months pregnant with her first baby. Accustomed to several running, cycling, swimming, and weight workouts every week, Evan anticipated that she'd have to cut back some. "I thought I might have to reduce my weekly mileage, but because I've known runners who've run through their pregnancies, and because I've been running since I was 18, I thought I would be comfortable with running all the way through," she explains. "That hasn't been the case."

One issue is the physical feeling of running with a belly. "I began to show right away," Evan says. "I went from concave to convex in two weeks. When I move, my belly moves independently of me now. It feels very weird." Evan is also concerned about potential long-term damage from putting excess stress on her ligaments and joints at a time when pregnancy hormones have relaxed these supporting structures. "Walking feels easier. Intuitively, it feels like the right thing to do to safely maintain strength and endurance that I'll need for labor and delivery."

Even at two months, Evan has noticed the shift in her center of gravity in other activities as well (she doesn't spend a lot of time sitting still). It's particularly apparent during swimming, yoga, and tai chi. "I feel like I'm swimming on a slightly inflated beach ball," she says. "And with yoga and tai chi, it's almost like I know intuitively what postures and positions to avoid." That's good advice for anybody.

Another obstacle has been unflagging nausea. "I'm nauseous from the minute I wake up until I go to sleep. I think it began at the moment of conception." Walking and swimming offer the only breaks that Evan gets from the tedium of constant queasiness. "I walk five miles, four times a week, swim one mile two or three times a week, and spin on my bike twice a week. Those are the only times I don't feel the nausea," she says. "It seems to have a lot to do with the movement." It's a huge struggle for her to get moving; even standing up can be a challenge. "I remind myself that I want to maintain as much of my pre-pregnancy fitness as possible so that I have some advantage during labor and so that it will be easier to get back in shape after delivery." Once moving, her stomach settles after 5 or 10 minutes, and she gets a 30-minute feel-good window after she's done, too, unless she has to get right back in the car.

Why walk or move at all when you feel so lousy? "I've enjoyed incredible good health because I exercise regularly, and I don't want to trade that. Pregnancy is not an illness, it's a physical challenge. My body is supporting me and my baby now, and I want to give it the best chance to keep all my systems working optimally."

Every Time You Exercise

If you're already active, most of these guidelines are second nature. If you're new to exercise, it won't take long to adopt them.

- Warm up. Our warm-up routine and five minutes of slow walking is an ideal way to prepare your body for a workout.

- Cool down. Let your heart rate gradually return to normal by slowing your pace for the last 5 to 10 minutes of your workout and finishing with a few easy stretches (see chapter 3 for some specific moves to warm up and cool down).

- Keep water handy. Drink before, during, and after your workout, and anytime you're hot and thirsty.

- Use the right gear. Supportive, well-cushioned footwear is even more important now that you're carrying extra weight. A supportive bra and stretchy clothing that wicks sweat and moisture will make you most comfortable. Chapter 2 has info on shoes; chapter 8 on clothing.

- Pay attention to how your body feels, and heed any symptoms or warning signs (see "Warning Signs to Stop Exercising" on page 32).

- Plan for the weather. Dress accordingly if the weather is hot and or humid, or cold. Avoid exercising in extreme conditions; plan workouts for the coolest times of day or exercise in air-conditioning. In cold or windy weather, walk into the wind first (before you get sweaty) and plan to walk home with the wind at your back to avoid a chill.

- Gauge the intensity of your workouts, and stick with moderate effort unless you've got your doctor's okay. Take the talk test, use the Rate of Perceived Exertion method, or wear a heart rate monitor (see "Am I Working Too Hard?" on page 10).

- Don't hold your breath. We're not kidding—it's easy to do, particularly during strengthening or stretching moves, without even realizing it. Keep a deep, relaxed breathing pattern.

- After stretching or doing strengthening exercises in a sitting or lying position, be sure to get up slowly. If you stand up quickly, you may feel dizzy or faint because the blood has quickly shifted away from your brain.

Take It from Us:

Walking through Nausea

"Lying on a couch has never been one of my favorite pastimes. But with my second pregnancy, nausea forced me to log some good time there for much of the first trimester. Except when I slept, I felt like an unwilling passenger on a lurching ship. I knew it was important to eat right to nourish the baby, but almost everything was tough to get down, and sometimes it just wouldn't stay. Eventually, I found some foods that I could stomach: Wendy's plain hamburgers, chocolate shakes, plain bagels, caffeine-free Coke, and orange soda topped the list. Not exactly a nutritionist's dream diet for pregnancy, but it helped, at least for an hour or so at a time.

"Another discovery: When nauseous, never take your prenatal vitamin in the morning, especially on an empty stomach. You're bound to see it again. And finally, though every fiber of your being seems to tell you to lie down, try to get out and walk. I found that I could handle 15 minutes, going very slowly, and would do a little trail loop that happened to be next door to my older daughters' preschool before I picked them up. I won't say it's a cure, but it was a welcome break from the tedium of feeling ill.

"Though the last thing you want to hear is, 'It should go away at the end of the first trimester'—believe me, no consolation when that's six weeks away—it's really true. The nausea really did gradually fade, and eventually leave for good."

—Tracy

GOOD QUESTION

Are there any foods that can help with pregnancy-related nausea, or at least give me enough energy to keep exercising?

A range of experienced, active moms indulged us in a survey of "Best Anti-Nausea Foods." Most agree you should listen to your cravings, in moderation. Your body may know more than your brain when it comes to nausea. Here's a brief summary of some favorite foods to soothe the savage gut:

- "Balsamic-vinegar-dressed salad at the end of dinner."

- "Medium-sized potato microwaved for four to six minutes (butter to taste)."

- "Just salt. Always. The more the better—stuff that disgusted me when I wasn't pregnant. Like 7-Eleven hot dogs. I would go in and get four of them at once. Gross, I know. I just couldn't get enough salt. Plus I had to keep my blood sugar up—especially after a workout. If it dropped too low then I had nausea."

- "It went downhill with each pregnancy: The first pregnancy, it was eight glasses of water a day and an organic salad at lunch. By the third pregnancy, it was chow down some Cheez Doodles on the run and wash them down with Diet Pepsi. Ugh."

- "Any food that wasn't green. Fruit—any and all."

- One husband wrote, "Crackers, saltines." The next day he wrote again: "Addendum—a debate has ensued: blueberry pie."

- "Salty pretzels with cream cheese and soda water."

- "My safest eating was in bed; I kept my prenatal vitamins, pre-peanut-buttered whole-wheat crackers, and water bottle by my bed. Before going to sleep I'd take half a vitamin, two crackers, and guzzle eight ounces of water and then I'd do the same as soon as I woke up before I got the urge to puke."

Bottom Line: Not surprisingly, experts recommend small portions of foods high in protein and complex carbohydrates taken often and with water, especially if you're tossing them occasionally throughout the day. Our panel's frequent mentions of lots of water, salty snacks (the salt may aid in palatability), fruit (complex carbohydrates), and some protein (peanut butter) don't fall far from the mark.

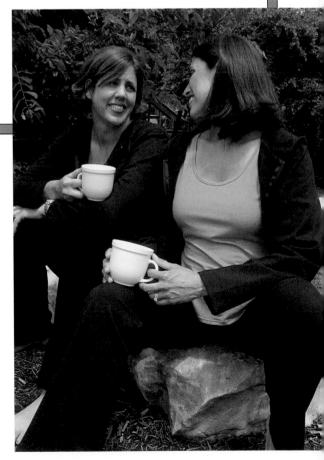

Treating Exercise Soreness

As you're working to maintain a pregnancy exercise routine, and especially if you're an experienced exerciser, you may run into the occasional sore or tight muscle. But your response may have to change now:

- Don't take any medication—prescription, over-the-counter, or even herbal—without checking with your doctor. (Of course, don't stop taking medications for a chronic condition such as asthma without checking with your practitioner first.)

- Specifically, don't take aspirin, ibuprofen (Advil, Motrin), or naproxen (Aleve) unless prescribed by your doctor. These may cause fetal bleeding. Tylenol or any other brand of acetaminophen is usually okay—but still ask the doc first.

- Don't sit in hot tubs or saunas. Excessive heat will raise your body temperature and can interfere with baby's development.

- Do stretch gently but regularly–ideally, after all exercise.

- Do get your partner to gently massage your feet, legs, back, and shoulders (try sitting straddling the back of a chair, leaning on a pillow, for a relaxing neck and shoulder rub) to improve your after-exercise comfort.

- Do use ice on sore spots (ankles, knees, muscles). Crush the ice in a plastic bag or moist towel, and rest on the sore area for up to 15 minutes.

Checklist: What the Doctor Wants to Know about Your Exercise Plans

Before the first prenatal visit, make sure you add exercise to the list of a zillion questions swirling in your head. This is a good chance to talk with your doctor about what's okay and what's not for your specific pregnancy, and with so much to think about, it helps to be prepared. Your practitioner may want to know the following:

- Do you exercise now?

- What activities do you do regularly?

- How often? Once or twice a week? Two to four times a week? More than four?

- For how long? Less than 20 minutes? About 30 minutes? 40 minutes or more?

- How intensely? Would you describe your effort as easy, moderate, or hard?

- Does your occupation involve walking, heavy lifting, or prolonged sitting or standing?

- If you've been sedentary, for how long?

- What are your goals and reasons for exercising?

- What activities and sports would you like to do while you're pregnant?

- Would this be different from what you're doing now?

- Are there medical reasons that have prevented you from being active in the past?

- Is this your first pregnancy? If not, how many pregnancies have you had?

- If you've been pregnant before, did you miscarry, or were there any complications that kept you from exercising then?

Am I Working Too Hard?

Almost any pregnant woman–especially a first-timer–will tell you that one of her biggest concerns about exercising is overdoing it. Since experts recommend that most women stick with moderate-intensity exercise during pregnancy, it's smart to be thinking about this. Thankfully, you have three reliable methods to make sure you don't push too hard, but will still get the maximum benefit from your exercise. Needless to say, when you're just starting out it's best to err on the cautious side–less intensity rather than more. But as you begin to feel comfortable with your pregnancy, you can work at least moderately hard to burn a few more calories and maintain your fitness. Here's how to be sure you're there.

EASY AND QUICK: THE TALK TEST

To maintain a moderate level of effort, you can work to the point of having noticeable breathing, yet still be able to maintain a conversation while you exercise. Conversing won't be quite as easy as if you were chatting side by side on a couch, but it shouldn't be a struggle and it shouldn't leave you breathless or gasping. This sounds simplistic, but it's actually based on the scientific Rate of Perceived Exertion method described next. The talk test is a pretty good indicator that you've elevated your heart rate and your body's demand for oxygen while staying at a safe, maintainable level of effort.

A BIT MORE THOUGHT: THE RATE OF PERCEIVED EXERTION (RPE)

The RPE is a fancy way to say that you simply compare how hard you feel you're working to a standard scale. It takes a little practice to rate yourself, but you'll quickly get the hang of it. Researchers originally developed the scale with ratings from 1 to 20, and corresponding word descriptions such as "very light" and "extremely hard." In practice, it's easier to use a simpler 1-to-10 scale (see the box), which many physiologists now also use. Interestingly, it's been shown in research to be a useful and surprisingly accurate way of measuring exercise effort, even compared to more technical indicators such as heart rate and oxygen consumption.

A 1 on the scale means your effort is very, very weak, almost nonexistent (think watching *The West Wing*, reading the lastest issue of *Child*). As you move toward 10, the numbers represent progressively higher levels of effort, and eventually a greater proportion of anaerobic energy. (That's the quick-burn energy our bodies have in relatively short supply; unlike aerobic energy, which we can produce for hours, anaerobic energy production is great for high-intensity activity, but only available for shorter bursts of effort.) A 3 might be barely walking at window-shopping pace; 5 is a brisk pace, walking purposefully to get somewhere. An RPE of 7 is hard enough that you could only sustain it for a while (say, 40 minutes or so), and 9 is downright pushing your speed limit. Level 10 is all-out—you barely feel you can go another 30 to 60 seconds without absolutely having to stop. With this scale in mind, while you're pregnant you'll generally shoot for 3 to 7 on the RPE scale during exercise—lower for longer walks or on days you don't feel as good; higher when you're feeling stronger, and for shorter, faster walks.

How can such a broad range on the scale (3 to 7) be safe? Because of the broad range of factors that influence effort. The more fit you were before pregnancy, the higher you can safely push your RPE during a walking workout. The shorter your walk, the higher the RPE you can maintain; the longer the walk, the lower the RPE. Even the conditions matter—walking over hills or on a hot day begs hanging at the low end of the RPE target range. A cool, comfortable walk on level ground allows for a higher RPE. As always, you have to use good judgment, and we recommend talking to your doctor and then practicing thinking about your RPE when exercising so you get to learn what's a 4 and what's a 6 on your own personal scale.

TIP:

The warm-up gets your blood flowing, increases the temperature of your muscles and joints making them more compliant and less injury prone.

Rate of Perceived Exertion (RPE) Scale

RPE	EFFORT
0	Nothing at all
1	Very, very weak
2	Very weak
3	**Moderate**
4	**Somewhat strong**
5	**Strong**
6	**Strong**
7	**Very strong**
8	Very strong
9	Very, very strong
10	Very, very strong; maximal

The 1-to-10 scale for Rating of Perceived Exertion (RPE). While you're pregnant, target exercise in the 3 to 7 range unless your doctor directs you otherwise.

The Gold Standard: Measure Your Heart Rate

Yes, you'll have to either take the time to actually check your heart rate while exercising, or buy or borrow a heart rate monitor and wear it to follow this method. But it's the most accurate measure of your exercise intensity, and it's surprisingly easy to learn.

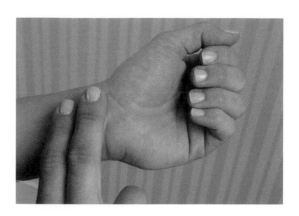

The simplest approach is to actually take your pulse for 10 seconds while exercising. You can feel it either at your wrist or your carotid artery (neck). For a wrist pulse, place two fingers from one hand on the inside of your other forearm, just below the wrist joint, more to the thumb side of the arm. For the carotid pulse, place two fingers on the side of your neck next to your throat, at about the height of your Adam's apple. Practice finding these before exercising, so you're comfortable and familiar with their location once you get out on a walk. After counting the pulse for 10 seconds, multiply by six to determine your

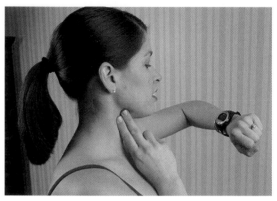

heart rate in beats per minute. The other option is to use a heart rate monitor (see chapter 2).

But what should your heart rate be when exercising? If you've used heart rate as an exercise guide before, you know that your target heart rate isn't a firm number but a zone that can range up to 15 beats per minute from lower to upper end. But be aware that different target ranges apply now, due to two factors. First, your resting heart rate is 10 to 15 beats per minute higher now that you're pregnant. (This happens because of the increase in blood volume in your body, and also possibly due to hormonal changes.) Second, even when exercising at higher intensity, women don't get their heart rates up to the same level during pregnancy. The best way to determine the right exercise intensity and heart rates for you is in a discussion with your health practitioner.

The accompanying box offers representative target heart rates, depending on your age. This is based on the simple fact that your target heart rate for exercise is estimated as a percentage of your *maximum* heart rate, and a person's maximum heart rate tends to drop with increasing age. The American College of Gynecologists and Obstetricians recommends that pregnant women participate in exercise at moderate levels, but it doesn't specify target zones. The four age-based zones here are recommended

Heart Smart Exercise: Modified Target Heart Rate Zones for Exercise during Pregnancy

Your Age	Target Heart Rate Zone	Pulse Count for 10 seconds (beats/minute)
Less than 20	140–155	23–26
20–29	135–150	22–25
30–39	130–145	21–24
40 or greater	125–140	20–23

Talk to your doctor to assure that these ranges are right for your pregnancy and circumstances.

by the Canadian Society for Exercise Physiology. If you're just starting an exercise program, stay at or below the lower end of the range for your age. You'll also want to stay at the lower end of the range later in pregnancy, when you'll naturally slow down. On the other hand, experienced and fit exercisers can work toward the upper end of the range, especially during shorter exercise bouts, while staying at the middle or lower end of the range during longer walks.

Bottom line: Talk to your health practitioner about the right target heart rate for you during pregnancy. Offer these ranges as a starting point for your consideration, but adjust according to your specific circumstances. Some of the women we interviewed who were very fit going into pregnancy got the okay from their physicians to work in a higher range. But it's important to discuss your circumstances with your doctor so that together you can make a decision based on your particular pregnancy and level of fitness.

GOOD QUESTION

Are there any exercises or activities I should avoid during pregnancy?

In general, stay away from abrupt movements that would jar you or the baby or stretch ligaments, and certainly avoid anything that causes discomfort or just doesn't feel right. Specifically, experts suggest staying away from the following moves:

- Deep knee bends, which put too much stress on knee joints, especially when you're carrying extra weight.

- Any moves that cause pulling or stretching on your belly, such as double leg lifts and full sit-ups; they're likely to cause back strain, as well as be just plain uncomfortable.

- Straight-leg toe touches—tough on the knee capsules and lower back.

- Lying on your back after week 20 of your pregnancy; this can cause faintness and dizziness, because the weight in your abdomen can block the flow of blood to your heart.

- Bouncing, jerky movements, or quick changes of direction. All can put lax joints at risk.

There are certainly a number of sports and activities to avoid during pregnancy. Any extreme sports, high-impact activities, or those with abrupt collisions are discouraged. We don't dare offer a complete list of such risky activities, as we're sure to leave something out (or offend someone who effectively did that activity until her ninth month without a hitch!). With that caveat, here's a small (and incomplete) sampling of activities to avoid. Use your best judgment (and a chat with your physician) if you have any doubts.

- Skydiving.

- Scuba diving.

- High diving. (In fact, we think anything with *diving* in it is a no-no.)

- Water polo.

- Horse polo. (Anything with *polo* in it, too, except maybe Marco Polo in the shallow end of the pool.)

- Ax throwing.

- Tree climbing.

- Log rolling. (All the lumberjack-contest activities can wait until after pregnancy, as well.)

- Contact sports.

- Martial arts.

- Anything with a moderate to high risk of falling, especially as your balance shifts.

Bottom Line: Activities that offer any risk of a hard impact, falling, sudden or jarring movements, bouncing or jerking, extreme movements for your joints (which are more susceptible to injury), or any compromise in your oxygen supply (obviously!) are all out. If you have any doubt about an activity, skip it. Pregnancy is only nine months, and you'll have plenty of time later to get back to a life of adventurous sports.

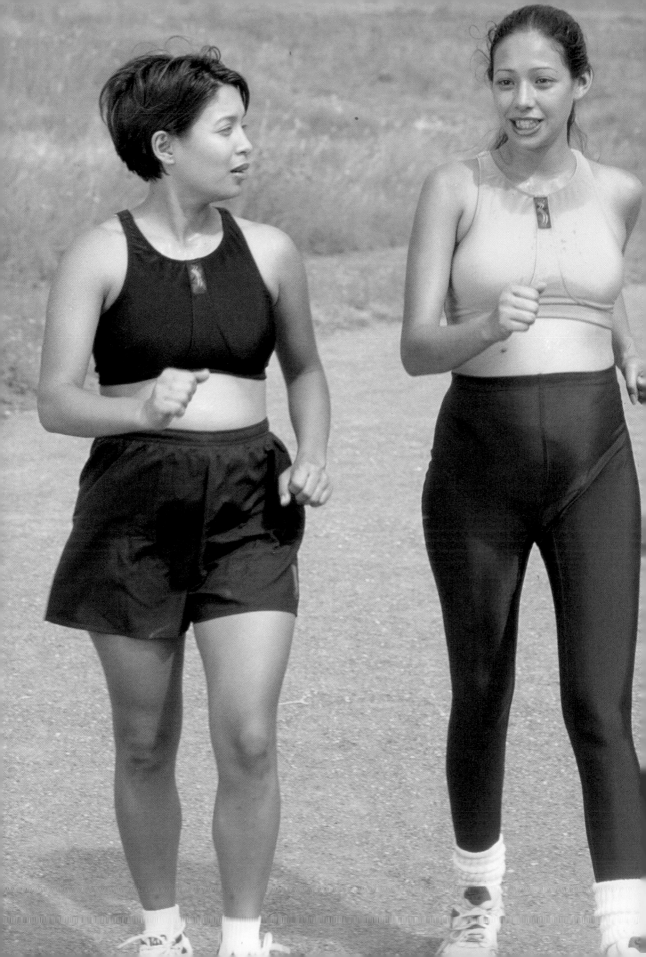

Gear 101: The Walking Basics

Gearing Up to Go

The beauty of walking is that it's so simple, you really don't need a bit of special equipment or preparation to make it a part of every day. Still, the beauty (or curse?) of twenty first century America is that there's plenty of gear out there for pregnant women (and others) leading an active lifestyle. And some of it is really fun, convenient, and even helpful. But we'll save most of it for future gear chapters. For now, let's focus on three essential items you may be considering (at least using, if not buying) as you get started walking regularly: walking shoes, a heart rate monitor, and a treadmill. We've got some pretty important tips for each of these.

It's Gotta Be the Shoes

The more you'll be walking, the more your shoes matter. And the faster you walk, the more you'll notice the difference between a walking shoe and other athletic styles (say, running or cross-training). But even a moderate stroll will be more comfy in shoes designed for the walking stride, especially as you gain weight and lose a bit of balance through your pregnancy. The walking gait is a distinctive motion of the foot as it rolls from heel to toe, and that leads to three simple reasons why any serious walker (consider yourself one, starting now) should be investing in true walking shoes.

First, fewer injuries. Walking shoes are designed for the unique heel-to-toe rolling motion of the foot in the walking stride—a stride distinct from running or other sports. Therefore, you're less likely to suffer discomfort or injury if you walk in walking shoes.

Second, greater durability. A shoe designed for walking is likely to hold up better for walking, just as a tennis shoe does better on the tennis court, and a running shoe is better for running. A walking shoe has the flexibility and support where you need it for walking.

Third, improved performance. A well-designed walking shoe can actually enhance your performance, by allowing a more fluid, rolling walking gait from heel strike to toe-off.

Four simple tests will help give you a sense of how well a shoe is designed for walking. Do them right in the store with salesclerks watching and maybe they'll learn something, too.

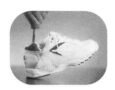

POKE TEST 1. A walking shoe should have a fairly low, rounded or beveled heel. This eases the transition as the heel first strikes the ground, and it allows the foot to roll from heel to toe gradually and smoothly, not abruptly. Push down firmly with a pencil at the very back of the shoe, inside the cup that surrounds the heel. If the heel is rounded or beveled sufficiently, the toes will lift off the ground.

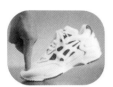

POKE TEST 2. The end of a smooth heel-to-toe roll is aided by a noticeable bend upward at the toe of the shoe, called toe spring. Push down on the end of the toe— the more the heel lifts off the surface, the more toe spring the shoe has. (The faster you walk, the more heel bevel and toe spring you'll appreciate in your shoes.)

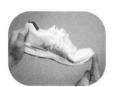

BEND 'EM. At the end of each stride, your foot bends through the ball just before you toe off. Grab the heel of the shoe firmly and push upward at the toes to see that the shoe bends where your foot naturally does, not under the arch. If the shoe does bend through the arch, stay away—that lack of support can lead to discomfort and even injury in the bottom of your foot and arch.

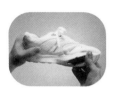

TWIST 'EM. As your foot accepts your weight, you imperceptibly load the outside of your foot first (the little toe) then shift your weight inward to the big toe. This slither from little toe to big happens quickly, without you even knowing it, but it's aided by a shoe with a bit of torsional flexibility. Grab the heel and toe of the shoe firmly and give a twist to look for modest flexibility so your foot's independent suspension can do its work.

Do I Need a Heart Rate Monitor?

If you're acutely concerned about not overstressing your own (and your baby's) cardiovascular system, but still want to be sure you get a decent workout, a heart rate monitor may be the thing to put your mind at ease. Your heart rate is the gold standard in assessing your exercise intensity, and a monitor can give you almost instantaneous feedback.

Heart rate monitors provide a shortcut for the old-fashioned method of placing your fingers on an artery and counting the beats per minute. Most are two-piece units. The monitor itself is a strap that's worn around the chest with two leads (flat, plastic areas) that rest below the breast or pectoral muscles. Some sports bras are made with a slot around the bottom band to hold a monitor. The heart rate signal is transmitted to a wrist receiver unit, which looks like an oversized digital watch. It displays your heart rate at the moment, in beats per minute. Some models also display other workout information and offer a variety of functions related to measuring, reporting, and recording your heart rate while you exercise. Basic models start at

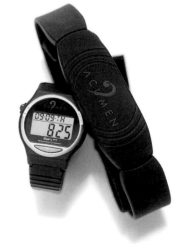

about $75; loaded models come with tons of bells and whistles that can shoot the price to more than $200. But most people don't need all the bells and whistles.

There are two features that you'll find especially handy now. One is the stopwatch feature, which means you can wear one device on your wrist but still monitor both heart rate and the length of your workout. The second is a target heart rate range with an alarm. This function lets you enter the lower and upper limits for your target heart rate (135 and 150 beats per minute, for example). On some models, you can set both a visual signal, such as a flashing bell, and an audible one that beeps when you go out of range. The advantage here is that you don't have to keep staring at your wrist to know when you've pushed too hard (or slacked off a bit).

If you're anxious about not overdoing it while you're pregnant, a heart rate monitor is a good investment. If you're not into gadgets, know that once you wear a monitor for a while, you're likely to learn to recognize when you're working and when you're not just by how it feels. Then you may be able to ditch the monitor and simply use the RPE method.

GOOD QUESTION

Can I Walk in Running Shoes?

In many stores, mention that you're a fairly serious walker or a pregnant women looking for a good supportive shoe for walking (or both), and they'll often steer you to a running shoe. Even some doctors, fitness experts, and coaches still recommend running shoes to serious walkers. We suspect they're harking back to their experience of years ago, when the term walking shoe meant stiff, all-white leather nurse's shoes that frankly would be lousy for actually trying to walk fast. But unless a physician or specialist is prescribing running shoes for a specific problem or pathology, a running shoe is actually the wrong call.

Nowadays the best athletic walking shoes are made with the same materials and manufacturing as the best running shoes—same cushioning foams, just as durable, just as supportive—but in a design better suited to the walking gait. The design differences boil down to three key things.

Difference 1. Your foot strikes the ground with only one to one-and-a-half times your body weight in walking, as opposed to a much more severe impact of three or four times body weight in running. So running shoes need lots more cushioning than walking shoes.

Difference 2. Your foot generally strikes the ground farther back on the heel (with the toes held higher up in the air) in the walking stride than in the running stride. The foot also rolls from heel to toe much more gradually in walking than in running.

Difference 3. A walker rolls farther off the toes at the end of each stride than a runner.

So a walking shoe should have a lower and more rounded or beveled heel than a running shoe. An extra-thick heel—needed to cushion high-impact running steps—only acts to lever the toes down quickly, which is bad for walking. In fact, a thick, squared-off running heel can even lead to shin soreness for a brisk walker, because as the toes slap down, the foot pulls on the shin muscles. If you're walking in running shoes and you notice burning or tightness in your shins, your first remedy is to change to walking shoes right away.

Walking shoes should also be more flexible through the ball of the foot than running shoes. Running shoes need cushioning up front, but sacrifice some flexibility in the process.

Bottom Line: Running and walking shoes are designed differently. Running shoes focus on shock absorption, with thicker cushioning in the heel and forefoot. Walking shoes are lower, more rounded in the heel, and more flexible up front for a rolling heel-to-toe stride. Make the switch to walking shoes, especially if you've been walking in running shoes and experiencing shin soreness.

Heart Rate Monitors-
Peace of Mind on Your Wrist

"I used a heart rate monitor throughout both of my pregnancies to ensure I did not go past the upper range of my target zone," says **Allison Librett,** a lawyer in **Atlanta, Georgia.** Her favorite features: the beep that alerted her when she went out of range, and tracker that tallied total minutes in her target heart rate range. Allison was able to adjust the band around her chest so that it stayed comfortable through the whole pregnancy.

Another approach is to use a monitor as a tool to help you learn what different levels of intensity feel like. Then you can wean yourself off it. "I used my husband's heart rate monitor for a few months until I got more comfortable with what the right pace felt like," says **Elizabeth McGuire of Austin, Texas.**

Walking Indoors: A World of Options

An admission first—we're not big fans of indoor walking. As a rule, we've all ventured out into even the coldest New England winters for our walks, and we feel that the fresh (if sometimes bracing) air brings benefits unrivaled indoors. Still, there are certainly valid reasons for occasionally not wanting to walk outside, and being pregnant is pretty high on the list. If it's especially cold, and in particular if snow and ice make footing dangerous, a walk indoors is a pretty levelheaded choice. Extremely hot weather can be equally unpleasant and even dangerous. The heavier and less fit you are, the more you may want to stay inside during extreme conditions.

A handful of other things may push your walk inside: safety concerns for a woman walking alone or traveling in an unfamiliar area, dangerous traffic and the lack of sidewalks or pathways, even the need to get in your walk while children are napping. Fortunately, if you do find yourself unable to walk outdoors, you have several options.

- **WALK THE MALL.** You may think mall walking is for the blue-haired set, but lots of malls open early, have active clubs, and even offer health screenings (blood pressure, cholesterol) and discounts for regular walkers. The real benefits, however, are safe, temperature-controlled settings and a reliably smooth walking surface—in larger malls, loops approach a mile in length. Check the hours at your local mall and see if it offers a formal program.

- **HEALTH CLUBS, YWCAS, COMMUNITY CENTERS, EVEN SKATING RINKS.** Many health and sports facilities have indoor tracks or walkways, sometimes surrounding courts or exercise rooms, or suspended above the gym floor.

- **CIVIC INSTITUTIONS: MUSEUMS, SCIENCE CENTERS, AQUARIUMS, ARBORETUMS.** Think about the kinds of places you'd spend a lot of time on your feet during a visit, and ask when they're least crowded (many offer discounts during off-peak hours). If you find one you like, consider a membership that includes free entry for the coming year—you and your new baby will both appreciate it!

- **DOWNTOWN WALKWAY OR TUNNEL NETWORKS.** City centers from Minneapolis to Des Moines,

GOOD QUESTION

Is Walking with Hand Weights a Good Idea?
Hand weights are often marketed as an easy way to add an upper-body punch to the cardiovascular workout of walking, but as a general rule we don't recommend using them, and that's especially true for pregnant women.

Hand weight promoters will tell you that to get the best workout, you have to bend your elbows and pump your arms vigorously, which is true. They'll add that if you maintain your walking speed, carrying hand weights can increase the calories you burn by anywhere from 10 to 50 percent. Independent research suggests that a 5 to 20 percent increase is more likely if you're carrying a reasonable amount of weight (less than 10 percent of your body weight). But keep in mind that this assumes you're not slowing down, which can happen quite easily with the weights in your hands. What promoters won't say is that you can probably get much of that same increase in energy expenditure simply by bending your arms 90 degrees and pumping them vigorously—without weights—during a brisk walk.

Also, hand weights bring with them concerns for people who have a history of shoulder or elbow problems or for anyone with heart trouble or high blood pressure. The latter is because the act of gripping the weights can boost your blood pressure somewhat artificially, an effect called the pressor response. This is exactly what you don't want to do to a pregnant body, and alone it's reason enough to stay away from walking with hand weights.

If you're considering hand weights to increase the aerobic intensity of your walks, you're better off simply focusing on walking faster. Use a technique where you maintain a tall, relaxed posture, bend your elbows so you have a quick, compact arm swing, and focus on increasing the speed rather than the length of your steps. If your goal is to build upper-body strength, you're not going to be able to safely and comfortably carry weights that are heavy enough to do that while walking anyway. (Three to five pounds is a likely upper limit.) For upper-body tone and fitness, you're far better off devoting 20 minutes to an efficient upper-body exercise routine after your walk several days a week (see our suggestions in "Trimester II").

If you really want a combination of aerobic boost and upper-body workout, consider using walking poles. It's all the rage in Finland—the land of cross-country skiers—and if you pole vigorously while walking, you can both boost the exercise intensity and get your upper body involved. Plus, you get increased stability on trails or unsteady footing—an important benefit late in pregnancy.

Bottom Line: Even if you walked with hand weights before pregnancy, leave them aside now. You don't want to risk increased exercise blood pressure or muscle or joint strain. Instead, spend a few minutes with weights after your walk for a quick upper-body

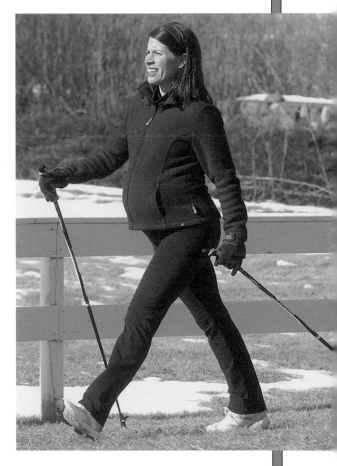

workout. If you do want to boost the intensity of your walk, simply pick up the pace. Bending your elbows and focusing on quicker steps will do the trick, and allow you to adjust your effort to how you feel. Or consider using walking poles for a combo aerobic and upper-body workout.

TIP:

Make sure there's a thumbnail width between your longest toe and the end of your shoe. It shouldn't slip at the heel or pinch anywhere.

and Rochester, Minnesota, to Rochester, New York, have constructed pedestrian bridges, covered walkways, and tunnels connecting downtown businesses, hotels, and civic centers. Some provide literally miles of safe, smooth walkways for your ambulatory exploration.

- **TREADMILLS.** Whether in your home or at a fitness center, a treadmill can be the perfect solution for anytime, any-weather walking.

TREADMILL WALKING: TRY BEFORE YOU BUY

If you've never walked on a treadmill before, be sure to try one before doling out the cash for a club membership or your own machine. Some people love treadmills and use them daily. Others never get comfortable with the idea of a moving surface and stationary scenery.

To be sure, try out a treadmill at a gym or a YMCA first. Most health clubs allow a complimentary visit if you're considering a membership; you may have to sit through the full sales pitch, but it's a good way to give a treadmill a whirl and see whether it's a setting you'd actually frequent. Or ask a friend if you can try hers for a couple of walks.

If you do decide to buy, look for the following features to make sure you get your money's worth. It'll be a bit more expensive, but it will also hold up through some serious abuse.

- You want a continuous-duty motor rated at 1.5 to 2.0 horsepower or more (2.0-plus if someone will be running on the machine).

- The belt should be at least 24 inches wide and 48 inches long, to avoid the *I'm-going-to-fall-off-the-back* feeling.

- Rollers should be at least two inches in diameter—the larger the rollers, the smoother the ride.

- Listen closely. The noisier the treadmill, the worse the workmanship and materials. If it drowns out the TV, that's a bad sign.

- Warranty. Expect a long one on the frame (lifetime is not uncommon) and at least two years on moving parts, motor, and electronics. You shouldn't have to buy an extended warranty (usually no bargain) to get these basics.

HOW TO STEP SAFELY ONTO A TREADMILL

Okay, an experienced treadmill walker may think this is silly. But the forward shift in your center of mass, combined with more lax ligaments and the fact that you don't want even the slightest risk of a fall, means that any pregnant treadmill walker—novice or experienced—should take care climbing on every time.

Fear not—treadmills are quite safe and easy to master. Here's how to step onto yours:

1. Begin by straddling the machine, with one foot firmly planted on the stationary part of the deck on either side of the belt, and hands on the handles.
2. Start the machine at a comfortable walking pace; not too slow, or it will feel unnatural to get on board. Try 2.0 to 2.5 mph.
3. Still holding the handles, paw the moving belt with just one foot several times, taking one-footed steps. Do the other foot a few times.
4. When you have a sense of the belt speed, step on with both feet and begin walking, still holding the handles. This is important: Look forward, not down at your feet. You'll want to look down, but don't; it can make you unsteady.
5. As you get used to looking forward, let go with one hand and let it swing normally. Then put it back and let the other hand swing free. Then only keep one hand very lightly on the handle, and finally let go entirely.
6. Stand tall, look forward, and use a natural walking technique. Don't look down to keep your feet on the belt—just use the handles in your peripheral vision to keep yourself centered and walking near the front of the machine.
7. When it's time to stop, put one hand on the handle and slow it to a saunter, then grab with both hands and straddle the machine before stopping it entirely. Step carefully when getting off the treadmill—it's normal to feel unsteady for your first few steps on solid ground.

TIP:

Always drink before you're thirsty. By the time you feel thirsty, you may have lost 1% of your body weight. A 2% loss can slow you down by 10% to 15% of your maximum potential.

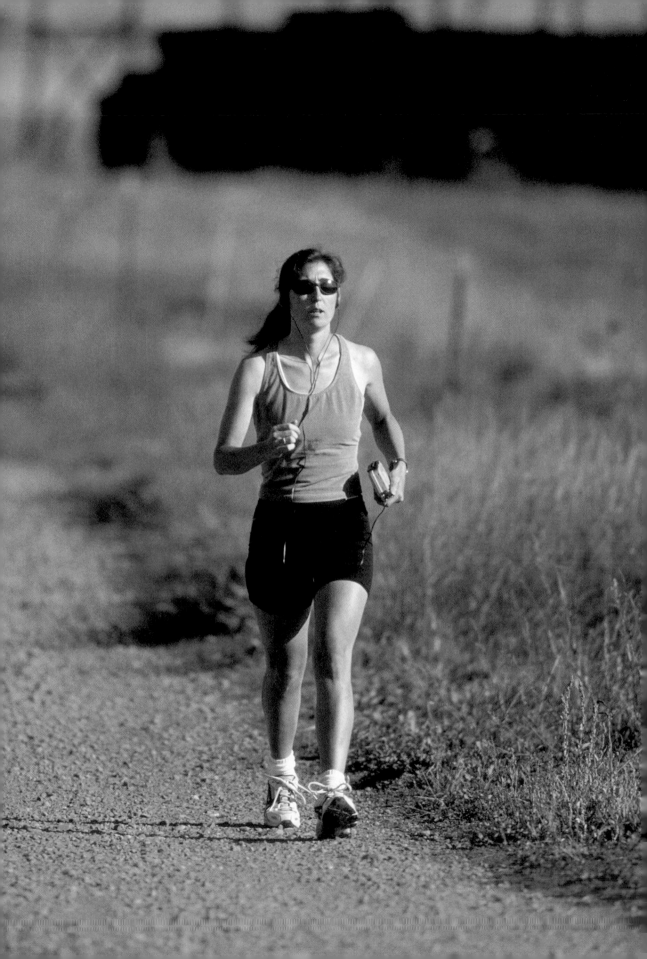

The Walking Program, Trimester I

3

Get Walking—Your Way

Researching and writing this book and creating our exercise recommendations has been a team effort for the three of us. And it's been an eye-opening process, even for the two-thirds of us who have already lived through the whole pregnancy thing. Mark expected some surprises, but even experienced, active moms Lisa and Tracy have found it enlightening. Here are some of the most interesting things we learned:

1. The medical profession is really behind the idea of exercise during pregnancy. Doctors don't just say, "Sure, go ahead if you want to." They really encourage pregnant women to be active. And they've done plenty of research on the topic—enough to be sure that for the vast majority of healthy women having "normal" pregnancies, routine physical activity is going to provide a pile of benefits that make it well worth the effort, with very little risk.

2. There are as many ways to make activity a part of your life, both during and after pregnancy, as there are women who have done it. Some walk once a day, early in the morning; some feel better taking multiple shorter walks. Some maintain an athlete's almost competitive mind-set—they're training for the big event. Others simply find physical and emotional relief in some daily activity.

3. Despite number 2, there do appear to be some universal truths: Social support helps; being flexible and listening to your body is important; consistency, but adjusting your expectations as your body and life change, is a key to success.

4. Another universal truth—walking works. Even when you're too nauseous, tired, emotionally fried, or feeling simply too gigantic to do much else, taking a walk—even a slow, relaxed, short one—tends to make you feel better.

These truths guide our recommendations, and should guide your walking throughout your pregnancy and beyond. But before giving you specific walking workout suggestions, we'll offer two other useful tools: warm-ups for before a walk, and stretches for afterward.

A Quick Walking Warm-Up Routine

Many assume that you only have to warm up if you're going out for an intense workout. Sure, the harder your intended exercise, the more you benefit from a warm-up. But even a gentle stroll will be easier if you've taken just a few minutes to increase the blood and oxygen flow to your muscles and slowly increased your joint and muscle temperature (hence the term *warm-up*) before starting. Given the changes your body is going through—discovering new ligaments and dramatically changing balance—a warm-up will also make you more comfortable and reduce the risk of injury, however short or long the walk.

Fortunately, walking is such an easy, natural movement that five simple moves can target the muscles that do most of the work. Make all the movements slow and controlled—nothing should feel like it jars or stretches anything. Do the routine standing up, resting a hand on something for balance (a nod to your shifting center of mass) on all but numbers 3 and 4. If you spend 20 to 30 seconds on each, the whole routine takes less than three minutes.

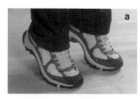

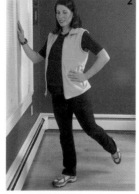

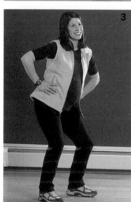

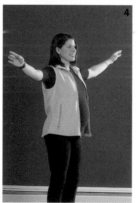

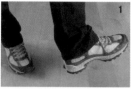

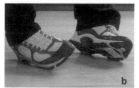

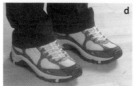

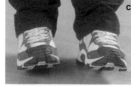

1 **Ankle circles.** (Loosens the shin, calf, and foot muscles.) Stand on one foot and lift the other off the ground. Slowly flex that ankle through its full range of motion, making a circle with the toes. Do six to eight in each direction on both feet.

2 **Leg swings.** (Warms muscles of the upper leg.) Stand on one leg and swing the other loosely from the hip, front to back. It should be a relaxed, unforced motion like the swinging of a pendulum, and your foot should swing no higher than a foot or so off the ground. Do 10 to 20 swings on each leg.

3 **Pelvic circles.** (Targets gluteal, hip, abdominal, and lower-back muscles.) Put your hands on your hips with your knees gently bent and feet shoulder width apart. Keep your body upright and make 10 slow, continuous circles with your hips, pushing them gently forward, to the left, back, and to the right. Then reverse directions and repeat.

4 **Arm circles.** (Warms shoulders, upper back, and chest.) Hold both arms straight out to the sides, making yourself a letter T. Make 10 to 12 slow backward circles with your hands, starting small and finishing with large circles, using your entire arm. Shake your arms out, then repeat with 10 to 12 forward circles.

5 **Up-side-back-downs.** (These are especially important if you experience shin soreness when walking.) Stand with both feet on the ground, about four inches apart. Then slowly roll your feet through four positions, holding each for a two-count:
Up: Stand up on your toes, heels high off the ground. (Stretches shins, works calves.)
Side: Stand on the outside edges of your feet, with the inner edges pulled upward.
Back: Stand back on your heels, with toes lifted high. (Stretches calves, works shins.)
Down. Return to both feet flat on the floor. Repeat the cycle 8 to 10 times.

Stretching—A Worthy Investment

As you age, your body's tissues gradually lose some of their natural elasticity—contributing not only to everyone's favorite result, sagging skin, but to stiffening muscles and joints, too. Regular exercise, while toning muscles, can also tighten soft tissues, further reducing flexibility. Add the hormonal and physical loads of pregnancy, and you've got a body that may literally make creaking sounds when you get out of the bed in the morning. Fortunately, research shows that even modest regular stretching can help stave off the natural and exercise-induced loss of flexibility, while likely reducing the chance of injury as well.

Coaches, therapists, and researchers agree that as little as a few minutes of stretching after every walk can help you maintain the full range of movement in your joints and stave off the stiffness that often comes with years of repetitive exercise. So at a minimum, get in the habit of doing the quick stretch routine after most walks: four simple stretches that take just four minutes. All are done standing up and are even easy enough to do in your work clothes after a commuting or lunchtime walk. Plus, stand-up stretches eliminate the need for what may become a true adventure late in pregnancy: getting down on the ground and back up again. Following that is a full flexibility routine—still ideal for a pregnant body, but it will take a few more minutes and provide more complete stretching for the whole body as well as some muscle toning. Use it when you have more time, or are feeling especially tight or stiff.

 TIP:

Anatomy of a walking workout: A four-minute warm-up before, a five-minute stretch afterward and whatever walking you can fit in between.

GOOD QUESTION

Is there any way to make sure my stretching is effective, and won't cause an injury?

Here are five rules for effective stretching:

1. Only stretch warm muscles. Stretching cold muscles can cause pain or injury, and won't be as effective as when muscles are more compliant. Many women find it easiest to make stretching an after-walk habit. But if you prefer stretching before your walk, at least do the warm-up routine (page 24) and walk easily for a few minutes before stretching. Our preference: Do the warm-up moves before a walk, and the stretches afterward.

2. Never bounce. Gently hold the stretch position for about 15 to 30 seconds—instead of counting, try taking five to seven slow deep breaths. Imagine exhaling muscle tension on each one.

3. Soften your knees. Pushing your knees straight can put a lot of strain behind the knee and on the lower back, so always keep your knees at least slightly bent.

4. Don't wince. Never push far enough that it causes discomfort; you should feel only a gentle stretch, but never any pain.

5. Rest a hand on something for standing stretches. This is especially important as you begin gaining weight and your balance shifts.

Bottom Line: Stretching should entail controlled, relaxed positions for all the major muscle groups; there should be no bouncing, and it should never hurt. To be effective, you should invest at least a few minutes almost every day.

This is called the *quick stretch* routine in the program charts and recommendations in this book. Do all of these stretches slowly, never to the point of discomfort; hold each stretch for six to eight slow, deep breaths. Begin each standing upright, resting a hand on something for balance whenever you need to. If you have time, go through the cycle twice.

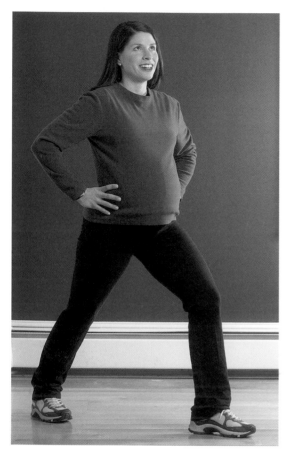

2 Back and hamstring. Stand with your feet together and your knees soft (not quite straightened). Move your left foot about 12 inches forward, lifting the toes and keeping the knee almost straight (but not locked). Bend the right knee a bit more and lean forward at the waist until you feel a gentle stretch in the back of the left thigh (hamstring). You may also feel this through the buttocks and into the lower back—keep your lower back flat, not excessively arched, throughout. Hold the stretch, then slowly stand up, switch sides, and repeat.

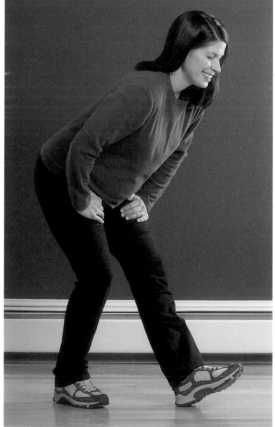

1 Calf/hip. Take a giant step forward with your left foot. Bend your left knee but don't push it beyond your left foot. Keep your right heel on the ground and your right leg straight behind you. Feel the stretch in your right calf. If you don't, then you need to take a larger step forward; if it's at all uncomfortable, take a smaller step. By gently contracting your stomach muscles, keeping your pelvis tucked under you (not tipped forward) and lower back flat (not arched), you'll also open up and feel a stretch in your right hip. Hold the stretch, then switch legs and repeat.

3a. Shin/thigh. Lift your right foot up behind you, reaching back to grasp your toes with whichever hand is easier and leaves the bent knee feeling most comfortable. Rest the other hand on something for balance, and keep your bent knee pointed toward the ground. Your heel doesn't have to reach your buttocks—just pull to the point of feeling a gentle stretch (but no pain) in the hip and thigh. By holding your toes rather than your ankle, you'll also get a mild stretch in the shin. Hold the stretch, then switch legs and repeat.

3b. Alternative hip/thigh. If you can't comfortably bring your leg up high enough for your hand to reach, instead do this "mini lunge" stretch: Take a medium step forward with your left foot. Bend your left knee but don't let it go beyond your left foot; keep your lower back flat and bend your right knee, allowing it to drop slightly toward the floor until you feel a stretch in your right hip and thigh. Hold the stretch, then switch legs and repeat.

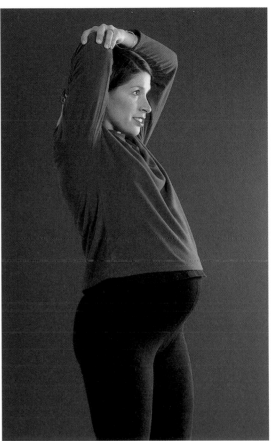

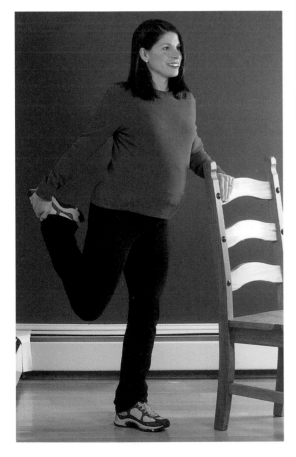

4 Shoulders/upper back. Point your right arm straight up at the ceiling. Then bend the elbow so your hand comes down behind your head. Reach up with your left hand and grab your right elbow, and pull gently to the left. Hold, then switch arms.

THE FULL FLEXIBILITY ROUTINE (FULL FLEX)

The four-minute after-walk stretch routine is great for a daily habit. But if you really want to minimize stiffness and discomfort, maintain a full range of motion in your joints, and even maintain muscle tone, it's worth investing a little more time in your stretching once in a while. The following full flexibility routine (called *full flex* in the program recommendations) takes a few more minutes, but is more complete and offers more strength work as you hold the stretch positions.

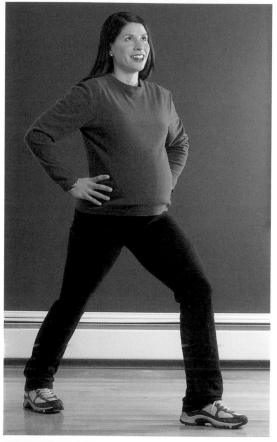

STANDING STRETCHES

1 **Calf/hip stretch.** (Same as the quick stretch routine.)

2 **Chest/front shoulder stretch.** Face a wall with your right arm raised, elbow bent at a right angle, and forearm and hand flat up against the wall. Now keep your arm in place but slowly rotate your body to the left, until you feel a stretch in the right chest and shoulder. Hold the stretch, then switch sides and repeat.

3 **Upper-back stretch.** Stand and raise your arms in front of you. Push your arms forward, rolling your shoulders forward and reaching as far as you can with your hands, feeling the stretch across the upper back. Hold, then relax and repeat.

4 **Lower-back stretch/pelvic tilt.** Stand with your back against a flat wall. Move your feet 10 inches from the wall, then bend your knees and tilt your pelvis beneath you, pushing your lower back against the wall. Gently tighten your abdominal muscles to hold this position. Hold for several slow deep breaths. Then stand up, relax, and repeat.

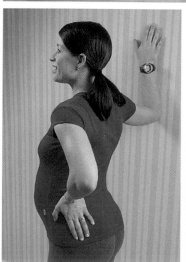

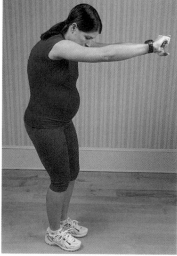

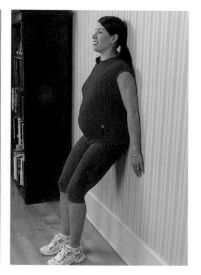

FLOOR STRETCHES

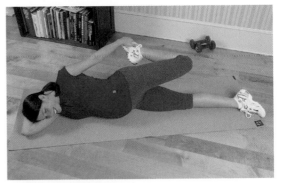

5 **Lying quadriceps/hip stretch.** Lie down on your right side, extending your right arm. Bend your left knee, bringing your foot behind you and grasping the toes with your left hand. Don't pull the foot to your buttocks, but just to the point of feeling a gentle stretch in your thigh and hip. Be careful not to arch your back on this stretch. Hold, then relax and do the outer thigh stretch (number 6). Switch sides and repeat.

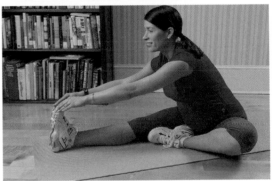

6 **Outer thigh stretch.** Lie on your right side. Without rolling your hips forward, place your left leg on the ground in front of you with the knee bent at a right angle. Feel the stretch in your outer thigh. For more stretch, you can extend your left leg straight. Hold, then switch sides and repeat stretches 5 and 6.

7 **Modified hurdler's stretch.** Sit with your right leg extended straight, your left knee bent, your left leg on the ground, and the bottom of your left foot alongside your right knee. Without locking your right knee (it can bend slightly), bend forward from the waist and reach toward your right foot. Try not to round your back—keep it flat—and only go to the point of a gentle stretch in the back of your thigh, but no pulling or discomfort. Hold, then switch sides and repeat.

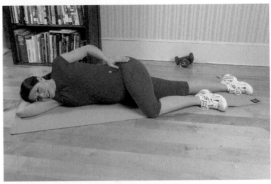

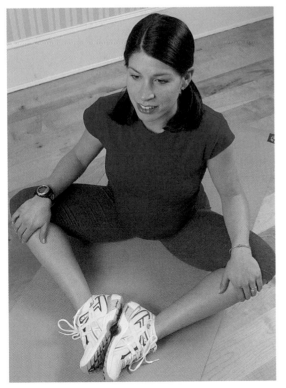

8 **Inner thigh stretch.** Sit with your knees bent and the bottoms of your feet together in front of you. Push your knees toward the floor to stretch your inner thighs (you can also put your hands on the ground behind you for support, and to avoid rounding your back). Hold, then relax and repeat.

TIP:

Go for a well-rounded workout: you use more of your body's 650 muscles and 208 bones when you walk than when you run.

The First-Trimester Walking Program

We'll give you exercise recommendations for each three-month period during your pregnancy (three trimesters) and the year after your baby's birth (four postmesters). The program is given for three levels, but don't feel locked into them—they're just a starting point as you set your own goals for daily and weekly exercise. And know that the suggestions are just that—suggestions. If your doctor wants you to do more walking or stretching or strengthening (or less), or if you're physically feeling more or less able, then obviously adjust accordingly. But whatever the level, let this program encourage you to make physical activity an absolutely routine part of your pregnancy.

GOOD QUESTION

What do I do to stay safe when out walking?

Most safety tips are pure common sense and hold for all walkers, pregnant or not. But you should think about all of these every time you head out to walk, until they become part of your walking habit.

1. Always walk on a sidewalk or path separate from the road when available. On the street, stay on the far left side, always facing oncoming traffic.

2. Carry identification and a cell phone or enough change to make a telephone call.

3. Know where you are and where you're going. Choose walking routes with "bail-out" opportunities—junctions where you can choose to do your full walk or take a shorter loop back to the start.

4. Seek routes with public bathrooms (or amply foliaged areas) along the way—inevitably, nature will call on a walk. It's a reality of the amazing compressed bladder.

5. Be aware that personal stereo headsets make you less aware of your surroundings, bicyclists, traffic, or an approaching stranger. Wear one if you must, but never in an unfamiliar area, and stay extra alert.

6. If you're approached by a loose scary dog, stay calm and try not to show fear. Say "no" and "go home" in a low, firm voice, but don't be threatening.

Back away slowly. Whether you have trouble or not, notify the police or animal control officer. If dogs are a problem on your walks, change routes or carry pepper spray.

7. Be highly visible when walking in the dark, and at dawn and dusk when visibility is deceptively poor.

For best results:

• Wear retro-reflective materials, not just light colors. Retro-refelectives bounce light back toward the source, making them highly visible in car lights.

• Get 360-degree coverage. Consider a reflective vest (available at most running stores).

• Carry a light. Many small LED flashlights and headlamps are featherweight and easy to carry, but throw enough light to be visible from hundreds of feet away.

Bottom Line: Walk in familiar areas, know your routes and alternatives, carry identification and a way to get in touch with a ride if needed (change, cell phone), stay on sidewalks or walk on the left, facing traffic, and be sure that you're very visible in reduced light.

THE STARTER QUIZ: HOW MUCH EXERCISE IS RIGHT FOR YOU?

That's a question that can really only be answered by you and your physician in consultation. But you can help your discussion along by taking this quiz first. If nothing else, it will give you something to talk about at your first visit. It should, however, help you consider both how active you've been and how ambitious your goals are. For each question, pick the answer closest to your situation, then tally up the score. The result will steer you toward a walking program (we call them *low-key*, *moderate*, and *challenging*) suited to your current fitness and goals. Then your doctor can weigh in on whether that's the right approach for you, and you can get walking.

1. How often did you get conscious exercise before getting pregnant?
   a. Once a week or less.
   b. Two to four times a week.
   c. More than four times a week.

2. How long did you typically exercise (not your longest workouts, but the average)?
   a. Less than 20 minutes.
   b. Usually 20 to 40 minutes.
   c. Usually 45 minutes or more.

3. How would you describe your effort for most of your exercise?
   a. I get no conscious exercise, or what I do is very easy and comfortable (say, walking at window-shopping speed or with a constantly sniffing dog, or very low-intensity yoga).
   b. Moderate (think brisk walking, bike riding on mostly level ground, recreational swimming).
   c. Hard (for example, fast walking, serious hiking, running, weight lifting, lap swimming, mountain biking, aerobics classes).

4. Aside from any conscious exercise you do, how active is your average day?
   a. Low-key. Unless you count walking to the car, mailbox, fridge, or short trips for errands, I'm either sitting or standing still (or snoozing) for much of the day.
   b. In gear. I'm often walking around at work, cruising up and down the stairs, or chasing kids (for example, an active nurse, teacher, or stay-at-home mom).
   c. Overdrive. I have a physically demanding job or lifestyle that really keeps me moving (think carpenter, river rafting guide, FedEx delivery person).

5. How fit were you pre-pregnancy: If you were helping a friend carry groceries up two flights of stairs, which best describes how it would go?
   a. I'd walk slowly, maybe take a break, and be breathing pretty hard by the time I got to the top. (Given the choice, I'd find an elevator!)
   b. My arms might get tired but I'd be able to walk up nonstop; I'd be breathing noticeably but in control.
   c. No problem: I'd carry two bags and move easily up the steps without giving it much thought.

6. What best describes your goals for exercise results during pregnancy?
   a. I want to stay healthy and be more physically ready for childbirth and keep my stress levels down.
   b. Same as (a), plus I'd like to avoid gaining any excess weight and maintain my muscle tone and flexibility during this pregnancy.
   c. Both (a) and (b), plus I hope to maintain my aerobic fitness, strength, and flexibility as much as physically possible, and bounce back quickly after delivery.

SCORE:
1 point for each (a), 2 for each (b), 3 for each (c).

People who are successful at exercising regularly tend to fit workouts into their existing schedules rather than changing their schedules to accommodate a workout.

IF YOU SCORED:

6–9 POINTS. You're best to start with the **low-key** program. It will help guide you to a modest daily activity habit without pushing too hard or adding stress to your days.

10–14 POINTS. Try the **moderate** program. If it feels too challenging in any way—too much time, or the walks are leaving you exhausted—back down to the **low-key** program. On the other hand, if you're feeling great but don't think you're getting enough exercise, gently ease up into the **challenging** program.

15–18 POINTS. Your current fitness and activity level suggests starting off with the **challenging** program. But if you have any stress or discomfort or just need a more restful week, then ease down to the **moderate** program; you can later work back up as your body responds.

Read through whichever program matches up with your score. If it sounds like you can handle it (and your doctor agrees), then get out for a walk. If not, chat with your practitioner, adjust down (or up) a notch if necessary, and embark on your agreed-to program.

GENERAL REMINDERS FOR TRIMESTER I

Begin by listening to your body. Some women will feel great, others miserable. And some days will be good, some bad. Let your feeling guide your effort.

But don't pass up walking. Despite the hormonal ups and downs you're due, don't skip your walks. You can go shorter, you can break it up, but walk every single day if possible.

Respond to your body. If you experience any of the warning signs outlined here, or anything feels wrong or discomfort persists, back off and check with your doctor right away.

Break up walks whenever you want. On days you're tired or don't feel good, don't be lulled into thinking that blowing off your walk is the right call. Sometimes a short walk (or two) can actually help. Get out the door just for five minutes, and see where it leads.

Start a warm-up and stretching habit. The easy warm-ups and after-walk stretch routines not only promote healthy joints and tissues, but provide a bit of resistance exercise as well. Adding some strength training is even reasonable now.

Warning Signs to Stop Exercising and Call Your Doctor

If you experience any of the following symptoms while you are exercising, stop and contact your practitioner right away:

- Dizzinesss or faintness.
- Chest pain.
- Increased shortness of breath.
- Irregular or rapid heartbeat.
- Calf pain or swelling.
- Difficulty walking.
- Uterine contractions that continue after you rest.
- Decreased fetal movement.
- Fluid gushing or leaking from your vagina.
- Vaginal bleeding.
- Pain.

Source: The American College of Obstetricians and Gynecologists

LOW-KEY PROGRAM (6–9 POINTS ON THE "HOW MUCH?" QUIZ)

Your first goal should be to build a fairly regular but modest walking habit. Because you may not have been especially active before pregnancy, this trimester isn't the time to become a superjock. There's too much going inside your body to add a new athletic goal to the mix. Instead, work on the basics of being just a bit more active. Figure out how and when you're going to fit walking into your day. Do you have child care for your older children? Can you walk before or during work? Can you find a friend to walk with—especially a pregnant friend who'll understand how you're feeling? You'll have a great trimester if you can get a walking habit started, along with quick prewalk warm-ups and postwalk stretches. Most of all, get your body and mind believing that you're a walker!

GOALS FOR A TYPICAL WEEK

▪ Begin walking at least three days a week. Over the first several weeks, add a fourth day of walking. During the next several weeks add a fifth day, so that roughly by week 10 you're walking five days a week (even if it's just 5 to 10 minutes on some days). The less you've done before pregnancy, the longer you can take to build up; the more you've done, the sooner you should get to five days of weekly walking.

▪ Add minutes slowly. Begin with 5- to 10-minute walks the first week or so. Gradually over the weeks, add a few minutes of walking every several days. By week 10, try to average two 20-minute walks and three 10- to 15-minute walks per week.

▪ Break your walks up if it helps. If you don't have the time or don't feel up to 20 minutes at once, then try two 10-minute walks instead (as seen, for example, on Saturday in the "Typical Week" chart).

▪ Do the simple warm-ups (page 24) before, and quick stretch routine (page 26) after, as many walks as possible.

A TYPICAL WEEK IN MID-TO LATE TRIMESTER I, LOW-KEY PROGRAM:							
	MON.	TUES.	WED.	THUR.	FRI.	SAT.	SUN.
WALK (minutes)	15	10	OFF	20	10	10, 10	OFF
OTHER STUFF	WARM-UPS, QUICK STRETCH	WARM-UPS, QUICK STRETCH		WARM-UPS, QUICK STRETCH		WARM-UPS, QUICK STRETCH	

MODERATE PROGRAM (10–14 POINTS ON THE "HOW MUCH?" QUIZ)

Your quiz score suggests that you get at least fairly regular, if inconsistent, exercise. Your goal should be to maintain what you've been doing and to simply build consistency this trimester. With all the physiological changes going on in your body, don't focus on building the duration or intensity of your workouts. Instead, get to the point that walking is truly a daily habit. You want to start finding regular routes of various lengths, and friends to walk those routes with you. Also, make the quick prewalk warm-ups and postwalk stretches a part of your walking habit.

GOALS FOR EACH WEEK

Begin walking at least four days a week. Over the first several weeks, add a fifth day of walking. During the next several weeks, add a sixth day whenever you feel up to it, so that by about week 10 you're averaging five to six days a week of walking (even if it's just 10 minutes on some days). The less you've done before pregnancy, the longer you can take to build up; the more you've done, the sooner you should get to a five- to six-day weekly average.

▪ Begin with 10- to 15-minute walks. After the first week, gradually add a few minutes on the days you feel good, building through 20- and then 30-minute daily walks. By week 10, try to average three 30- to 40-minute walks and three 15- to 25-minute walks per week.

▪ Break your walks up if it helps. If 40 minutes all at once isn't going to happen, then try 25 minutes now and 15 minutes later (as seen, for example, on Wednesday in the "Typical Week" chart).

▪ Do the simple warm-ups (page 24) before, and quick stretch routine (page 26) after, as many walks as possible.

▪ Midtrimester, add the full flexibility routine (not just the quick stretches) when you have time after walking; shoot for twice a week.

A TYPICAL WEEK IN MID-LATE TRIMESTER I, MODERATE PROGRAM:							
	MON.	TUES.	WED.	THUR.	FRI.	SAT.	SUN.
WALK (minutes)	40	25	20, 15	15	30	40	OFF
OTHER STUFF	WARM-UPS, QUICK STRETCH	WARM-UPS, FULL FLEX	WARM-UPS, QUICK STRETCH		WARM-UPS, FULL FLEX	WARM-UPS, QUICK STRETCH	

CHALLENGING PROGRAM (15–18 POINTS ON THE "HOW MUCH?" QUIZ)

With 15 points or more on the quiz, you're likely to already have quite a regular exercise habit. Plus, you may get lots of routine activity in daily life. So you can start off with a moderately challenging program of walking during pregnancy that's similar to what you've already been doing. There's no evidence that you have to cut back dramatically simply because you're pregnant (unless you have cause for concern; see "When to Back Off Exercise" on page 46). Indeed, even if you were doing a more jarring activity before pregnancy, you may be able to stay near your pre-pregnancy exercise duration and intensity simply by switching to low-impact walking.

That said, it's likely that the hormonal dance and physiological effort your body is going through will cause you to have some days when exercise is just like before pregnancy, and some days when it's anything but. The trick is to listen to your body, have great workouts when you feel up to it, and simply back off when you don't. The beauty of walking is that adjusting is easy to do, even midworkout. (That's why you bring a cell phone or plan flexible routes—what starts as an ambitious hour-long walk can be slowed down and end with a shortcut home if your body revolts.)

GOALS FOR EACH WEEK

▪ Begin walking five days a week. Initially, consistency is more important than duration or intensity. So over the first several weeks, add a sixth day of walking whenever possible, building to a regular six-day-a-week walking habit by about week 10 (even if it's just 15 minutes on some days). The less you've done before pregnancy, the longer you can take to build up; the more you've done, the sooner you should get to a five- to six-day weekly average.

▪ Begin with 10- to 25-minute walks. After the first week, gradually add a few minutes on the days you feel good, building through 30- and then 45-minute daily walks. By week 10, try to average three 40- to 60-minute walks and three 20- to 40-minute walks per week.

▪ Break your walks up if it helps. If 45 minutes all at once isn't going to happen, then try 15 minutes now and 30 minutes later (as seen, for example, on Wednesday in the "Typical Week" chart).

▪ Do the simple warm-ups (page 24) before, and full stretch routine (page 28) after, as many walks as possible.

▪ If you've been regularly lifting weights, keep it up but at a lower intensity and with safety modifications. If not, in Trimester II add the simple strength routine shown there. (See chapter 6, "Is It Time to Hit the Weights?")

A TYPICAL WEEK IN MID-TO LATE TRIMESTER I, CHALLENGING PROGRAM:							
	MON.	**TUES.**	**WED.**	**THUR.**	**FRI.**	**SAT.**	**SUN.**
WALK (minutes)	45	25	20, 30	35	25	60	OFF
OTHER STUFF	WARM-UPS, FULL FLEX	WARM-UPS, QUICK STRETCH	WARM-UPS, FULL FLEX	WARM-UPS, QUICK STRETCH	WARM-UPS, FULL FLEX	WARM-UPS, FULL FLEX	

Keep an Exercise Diary

Though it may seem like just one more thing on the already too-long "to-do" list, it's well worth getting in the habit of keeping an exercise log. It's a small investment in time and energy, for a big payoff. The investment: Write in your log for literally one minute every evening before bed, and look back over it for just a few more minutes every week or so. The payoff: Research and clinical studies show that people who keep an activity diary are likely to be more successful and stick with their exercise over time. There are several ways this probably works.

First, everyone likes positive feedback, and a diary makes your walking accomplishments concrete. ("Holy cow, I've walked 40 miles this month!")

Second, you can learn things from a log that make you a better, or at least smarter, exerciser. Note how you feel and what time of day you walk, and it may help you figure out what walk times best help stem nausea. Record where you walk, and figure out the loops you enjoy most. Jot down your stretches and you'll know what makes your back feel best.

Third, a log is a great planning and goal-setting tool. You can look a week (or more) ahead and anticipate when you'll be busy and when you'll have more time, and actually schedule workouts. In our log, there's even a "Goals" column to write anything from the number of minutes you plan to walk to whom you'll meet for a walk and when.

Last but far from least, there's a simple guilt effect—after all, who wants to see three zeroes in a row in the "Minutes Walked" column? Get in the habit of keeping a simple exercise diary. Either copy the log page in this book or get a calendar, and use it every day. It's guaranteed to make you a more successful walker.

TIPS FOR AN EXERCISE LOG

- **KEEP IT ACCESSIBLE.** On your nightstand, in your purse, on your desk at work—wherever you're certain to see it every day and always know where to find it.

- **MAKE IT EASY TO USE.**
  Write in this book, photocopy the log pages, or get a simple date book or calendar—whatever is easiest. Have a system—always write how far you walked in one place, how you felt in another, so it's easy to look back and find things.

- **WRITE *SOMETHING* EVERY DAY.**
  Don't skip days, or you'll forget what you did. Even if you did nothing, record it (and why not). Sometimes a few "zeroes" can be a motivator.

- **BUT DON'T WRITE TOO MUCH.**
  Specifically, no more than you're likely to be interested in reading later. Certainly how far you walked and how you felt—it helps you measure your progress. But over time, try to notice what's helpful and what's not. (Note your most comfortable shoes, stretches that help, favorite loops.)

- **LOOK BACK AT YOUR LOG ONCE IN A WHILE.**
  One goal of a log is to help you learn from your experience. Note places or routes you've enjoyed, exercises that are uncomfortable, or food that doesn't sit well on a long walk. Then glance back now and then to learn from these notes.

WEEK ONE:

Day	Goals	Miles/minutes, when & where?	Stretch? Strength? Other?	How are you feeling? Comments?
Sunday				
Monday				
Tuesday				
Wednesday				
Thursday				
Friday				
Saturday				

WEEK TWO:

Day	Goals	Miles/minutes, when & where?	Stretch? Strength? Other?	How are you feeling? Comments?
Sunday				
Monday				
Tuesday				
Wednesday				
Thursday				
Friday				
Saturday				

sample exercise diary

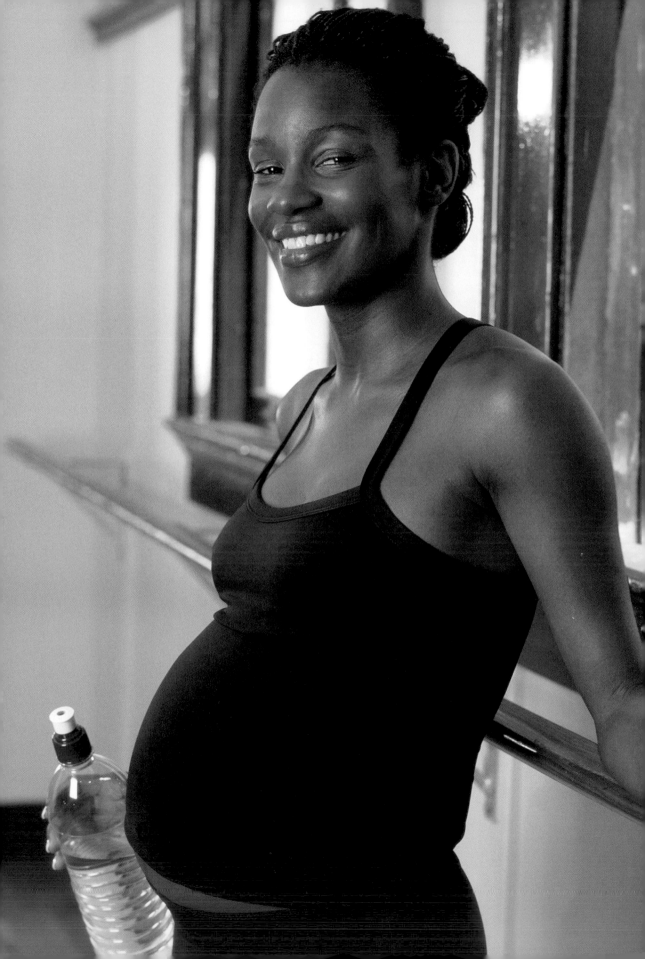

Moving Through the "Feel Good" Trimester

Time to Boost Your Walking

This second trimester is for many women the best part of their pregnancy. The not-so-fun symptoms that plague many women in the first trimester—fatigue, nausea, and the like—typically ease up, and labor and delivery are still far enough off to keep anxiety to a minimum. This time when you feel your pregnant-best is also the point when the exercise risk for baby is at its lowest. So if you've been waiting to step up your program or been held back by an unsettled stomach or the overwhelming urge to nap, this is prime time to make gradual, well-planned progressions in your exercise effort.

Along with a calmer stomach and more zip in your step, you're probably beginning to enjoy the pregnant look. Now that you've gained some weight and will continue to do so, it's important to think about the effects of this on your posture in general and especially as you exercise. It's also time to be careful not to let healthy weight gain get out of hand, simply by maintaining a healthy diet (sure, answer the wild craving now and then) and staying active.

KEYS TO SECOND-TRIMESTER SUCCESS

Even though this can a be a great time to boost your activity along with your increasing energy levels, it's still important to show good judgment and listen to your body. "Most women can continue whatever exercise regimen they like without harm to the pregnancy," says Marjorie C. Meyer, MD, associate professor of obstetrics and gynecology at the University of Vermont School of Medicine. "If at some time during pregnancy an exercise becomes uncomfortable—which is likely, eventually—that's the clue to decrease intensity or change the exercise." With this in mind, here are some rules for boosting your walking in the second trimester:

- **GREEN LIGHT, GO.** Provided your pregnancy is progressing normally and you're feeling good, this is the time to at least maintain, but ideally build your level of activity very gradually. You can take longer walks now and then, and pick up the pace on some of your shorter ones.

- **TALK TO THE DOC.** If you've had previous pregnancies in which you've gone into early labor or where the baby hasn't grown adequately, you must give your physician accurate and frequent updates on your activity level and how you're feeling. It may be you'll have to actually cut down on exercise in the second and third trimesters for the baby's and your own safety.

- **BUT DON'T BE A HEAD CASE.** It's not the time to worry that exercise is selfish because it's good for you, but bad for the baby. Dr. Meyer puts it succinctly: "For most women, if you are comfortable, the baby is comfortable."

- **STAY OFF YOUR BACK.** After the first trimester, the extra weight from baby may limit or block the flow of blood to major vessels and limit circulation when you're lying on your back. To prevent this, don't lie on your back after first trimester. Exercises such as abdominal crunches or pelvic tilts that you'd normally do on your back should be done on your side, on all fours, or standing.

- **STAY TALL.** Easier said than done, as you put on weight in your belly and breasts and your center of gravity shifts forward. Even if you had the posture of a prima ballerina before you were pregnant, the extra weight now can cause a more pronounced arch in your lower back: tilt your pelvis forward, and roll your shoulders forward. To counter this, do regular posture checks to make sure your pelvis is aligned properly, and build in time for regular strengtheners and stretches that can keep muscles ready to hold your body in its ideal position.

KEGELS FOR PREGNANCY

Pregnancy may be your introduction to an exercise called Kegels. Named for an American gynecologist, this move was designed to strengthen the muscles of the pelvic floor (the area around the anus and vagina) for stronger bladder control. Though for some women Kegels are about as interesting as flossing teeth and doing abdominal crunches, there's good reason to make them a regular practice. Keep these muscles strong, and you'll be less susceptible to urinary leaks late in pregnancy, when baby is large enough to press on your bladder. Another plus: Having a strong pelvic floor decreases the chance that you'll need an episiotomy during delivery. Once the baby's born, Kegels will still be important, this time to promote healing, tighten the vagina, and prevent incontinence.

To do Kegels, just contract and relax the pelvic floor muscles. At first, you might have trouble figuring out which muscles are the right ones. Head to the bathroom. You know you've zeroed in properly when you can stop the flow of urine. Hold the contraction for 10 seconds, then release and repeat. Once you get the hang of it, you can do Kegels almost anywhere—talking on the phone, waiting at a red light—and you can be sitting, standing, or lying down.

The goal? Do 10 to 20 Kegels three times a day, every day.

How Big Is Baby, Trimester II?

By the end of the second trimester, baby is about 14 inches long and weighs approximately two pounds.

Key developments: Organs continue to develop and function, fetal growth starts to pick up pace, and baby begins to move, kick (you'll feel this between 16 and 20 weeks), sleep and wake, and even hear your voice.

What this means for you: As baby grows more rapidly, your belly will start expanding more noticeably. This may lead to aches along your sides, caused by stretching in the ligaments that support the uterus. It's also time to switch to roomier clothing. Be aware that your center of balance is starting to shift. Expect an appetite surge (if you head out for a long walk, don't leave on an empty stomach). Though you'll begin to feel little kicks, they probably won't yet be strong enough to disrupt sleep. This is likely when you'll be feeling best, so it makes sense that it will also be your most active phase of pregnancy.

GOOD QUESTION

After losing my lunch for 12 weeks, I suddenly feel like dancing. What activities can I try with this newfound energy?

Our survey of active moms showed an inspiring array of activities they enjoyed doing during the second-trimester high, from the mundane to the magnificent. Some may be a bit adventurous for your tastes, but they should remind you that this is not couch-potato time. Anything that's safe and that you enjoy is fair game!

- "Walking laps in the parking lot at lunch hour (to stretch out my legs) and walking the dog every day after work."

- "I loved the weightlessness of swimming late in pregnancy . . . but didn't like the unsteadiness in the ocean."

- "A pedicure (just to feel good) and continued ballet every day; I could still do a full split on delivery day—Whoohee!"

- "Enjoyed both swimming and walking during second trimester. First trimester I was really tired so it was hard, and third trimester walking got less fun and swimming got more difficult so I had to slow down. But swimming was still a relief for my back."

- "Stadium walking; lived in Chicago near De Paul gym and basketball center so did the stairs."

- "Daydreaming while pregnant with Kacey (child one); chasing Kacey while pregnant with the twins (two and three)."

- "I don't think I know you well enough to tell you about my most enjoyable physical activity during pregnancy."

- "Again a de-evolution, from first pregnancy to third. First, worked out three to four times a week, mostly the stationary bicycle (until my legs really starting hitting my belly) or treadmill. For the second and third, the physical activity was chasing around the toddler(s), and shallow breathing when overwhelmed. . . ."

- "I would love someone to tote up the muscles used and the calories expended by taking care of very young children 24/7. It's not traditional exercise but it's an active lifestyle nonetheless!"

- "Ballet: No grand jetés after seven months, but the stretches and barré exercises were particularly helpful in so many ways (three pushes for each kid). Of course, the body changes of pregnancy gave me perfect 'turnout.' Only time I still felt graceful."

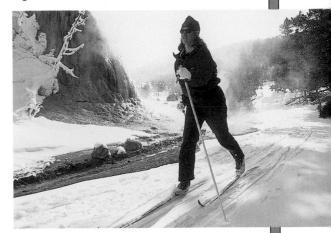

And the winner of the most adventurous pregnant undertaking award is Wendy Sharp, mother of three:

- "Depended on where we lived. I ran with the first one (once you got used to the urine running down your leg during the run, it wasn't so bad) in Arizona. I walked with the second—still Arizona, but that time running didn't feel so great. With third, we were in Michigan (with water and snow!) so I cross-country skied and then sea kayaked. The kayaking was really good. I mostly did it in my third trimester (summer). I even did a four-day Isle Royale kayaking trip with backcountry camping, no roads, 40 miles by water or air from a hospital—at seven months. (I kayaked the day he was born.) At the time I had a boat with a big cockpit so fitting in it wasn't a problem even though I was just huge in front—looked like a weasel taped to a basketball. But it felt so good to get off my feet and the kayaking position was perfect. My legs and crotch didn't ache—it just felt good."

Bottom Line: One trend—moms universally preferred low-impact activities (walking, stair climbing, swimming, cycling, Nordic skiing), and many chose things familiar from before pregnancy (ballet, kayaking). Many also recognized chasing older kids as plenty of work, and not one let being pregnant force her into dormancy—all really kept moving.

Great Foods for Pregnancy

The sometimes wild cravings of pregnant moms notwithstanding, there's plenty of healthy stuff that's both a pleasure to eat and especially good for you and the baby you're building. Here are some of the key nutrients you want to get in your diet. Some keep your system running well even with your high activity levels; others are crucial building blocks for baby.

KEY NUTRIENTS FOR A HEALTHY PREGNANCY		
WHAT	**WHY**	**WHERE**
FOLATE (FOLIC ACID IS THE HUMAN-MADE FORM)	Helps protect baby against neural-tube defects such as spinal bifida. Fights off anemia in Mom.	Broccoli, dark leafy greens. Cereals, lentils, breads.
PHYTOCHEMICALS	Act as antioxidants that rid body of cell damaging free radicals.	Most berries, broccoli.
OMEGA-3 FATTY ACIDS	Key for baby brain building.	Tuna fish, salmon, cod, haddock.
MOUTH-ACID NEUTRALIZERS	Thwart dental decay and gingivitis, which can lead to premature delivery.	Cheese.
CHOLINE	Good for memory.	Lean beef, eggs.
FIBER	Helps prevent constipation and hemorrhoids.	Bran cereals, oats, barley.
VITAMIN C	Helps protect body from oxidation damage, promotes strong bones and teeth, boosts immunity, increases iron absorption from food.	Citrus fruits, tomatoes, kiwi, mangoes, broccoli.
IRON	Prevents anemia, ferries oxygen to baby, can protect against low birth weight.	Liver, beef, seafood, dark leafy greens.
MAGNESIUM	Helps ensure strong bones and a healthy nervous system.	Sunflower seeds, spinach, wild rice, tofu.
VITAMIN B12	Helps carry oxygen and other nutrients to baby.	Red meat, fish, poultry, eggs, dairy products.
CALCIUM	Crucial bone builder; may help prevent pregnancy-induced high blood pressure.	Plain yogurt, dairy products, tofu, dark leafy greens, cereals.

FOODS TO ADD TO THE MENU . . .

Want an easy way to build some of the healthy nutrients above into your diet? Try some of these simple menu additions and savory snacks suggested by Elizabeth Ward, MS, RD, author of *Healthy Foods, Healthy Kids: A Complete Guide to Nutrition for Children from Birth to Six Years Old* (Adams Media, 2002):

- Hummus or cottage cheese and baby carrots or cherry tomatoes; whole-grain crackers: provides fiber, protein, beta-carotene (carrots), vitamin C, and lycopene (tomatoes); calcium in cottage cheese.

- ¼ cup roasted almonds: provides healthy fats, protein, vitamin E, magnesium, calcium.

- Yogurt parfait: Layer ½ cup low-fat yogurt with ¼ cup crunchy whole-grain cereal and ½ cup chopped fruit. Provides calcium, B vitamins, fiber, phytochemicals, vitamins A and C.

- Fruit smoothie: Mix 1 cup low-fat milk in a blender with a banana, 2 ice cubes, and 1 teaspoon vanilla extract. Blend until smooth. Provides calcium, B vitamins, fiber, phytochemicals, vitamins A and C.

- Celery filled with peanut butter; 8 ounces low-fat milk. Provides fiber, phytochemicals, folate (peanut butter), protein, healthy fat.

- ¼ to ⅓ cup tuna fish salad with whole-grain crackers: omega-3 fatty acids, protein, fiber, B vitamins.

- Hard-boiled egg and 1 ounce whole-grain roll: choline, an array of vitamins and minerals (from the egg); fiber and B vitamins from the roll.

Take It from Us:
You can do just about anything when pregnant.

"Lisa and I were sitting in a double kayak, taking instructions from the trip guide along with five other pairs of paddlers. We'd just finished an all-day paddle along 17 miles of the pristine northern shoreline of Kauai, Hawaii, and were about to beach in fairly high surf. The leader told us it was "routine," but spent a lot of time detailing how he'd land first, then use arm signals to direct us as to exactly how and when to come ashore and not get tumbled in the breaking waves.

"We're pretty experienced kayakers and wouldn't normally have given it a thought, except that Lisa was five months pregnant at the time. She sat up front, and the beauty of the double kayak was that all day she could paddle when she wanted or simply rest or stretch her back when she felt like it, while I happily toiled away in back. Normally called a divorce boat because of the need to paddle in synchrony, and the inherent risk to matrimonial bliss ('I said, left. No, no, the other left! Are you listening?'), we'd had a great day. Perhaps because I was extra deferential, and she was just enjoying being active yet physically so comfortable, the only trick had been her frequent trips overboard to respond to nature's call. (Kayaking may be extra-compressive to an already squeezed bladder.)

"As we paddled into position to go ashore, working to ride the backs of waves rather than surf in on the front of one and risk an abrupt and ungainly crash, we remembered the guide's final instruction: 'And when I go like this, just paddle straight in like you really mean it. No screwing around.' We lined up, timed the waves, got the

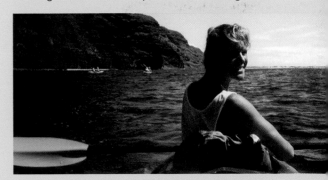

signal, and I saw a burst of paddling power like I hadn't felt all day—my wife had become an Evinrude motor! The kayak shot forward, rode the smooth water following a wave, and we glided well up the beach in a perfect landing. Lisa stepped daintily out with a wide grin of relief, and I thought what a great mom she was going to be if she had those reserves of strength to call on whenever her child would need them. And it's proven to be the case— she's the model of strength and self-reliance, a pattern she established long before the chidren were even born."

—*Mark*

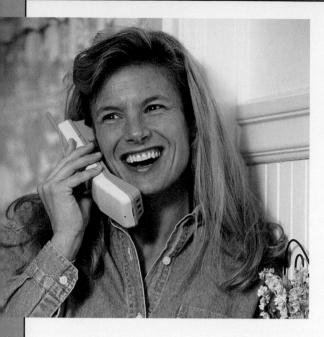

It Must Be in Their Genes

Sisters Larah Walker, 33, Tucson, Arizona; Lochen Wood, 29, Rifle, Colorado; and Lindsay Rosenthal, 26, Eden Prairie, Minnesota

Larah Walker, Lochen Wood, and Lindsay Rosenthal may live far apart, but that doesn't prevent a continual dialogue of questions, advice, and support from flowing among these three sisters. Larah, 33, has three boys, 2, 4, and 7, and lives in Tucson. Lochen, 29, in western Colorado, had just had her first, and Lindsay, 26, outside Minneapolis, was pregnant for the first time when we spoke to them. They grew up in an active family, where walking and sports were part of the daily landscape. "My mom has the attitude that if it's a mile away or less, walking is as easy as driving," explains Lindsay. Back in their hometown of Austin, Texas, Mom walks at lunchtime most days plus a few nights a week, and in Washington, DC, their grandmother walks daily and does errands by foot at age 84. This active heritage encouraged the sisters to stay active as adults, into their pregnancies, and—in Larah's case—beyond.

Building in Support for Exercise

As the veteran sister, Larah fields all sorts of questions, from whether to run or walk during pregnancy, to *Is it normal if my body feels this?* She's comfortable with all of them, having stayed fit through her first pregnancy, and then mastered the juggling act of finding time to exercise with one, two, and even three little ones to care for. The key has been to adapt as the family grew and needs changed, so she's done everything from early-morning walks, to outings with the single and double joggers, to finding a gym with outstanding child care. Currently, Larah goes to a nearby gym three mornings a week and fits in a run on the weekend when her husband can help with the boys. "Exercise keeps me sane. It burns off my nervous energy so I can concentrate on what really needs to be done instead of freaking out about the little things," she says. "On days that I go to the gym, it's also social time to talk about kid and mom issues with other moms, and if I'm alone, time to think."

With her first baby, she had the good fortune to have a friend right down the street, also pregnant. Both moms delivered within two weeks of each other, and they met every morning to walk. "It was a lifesaver, because on some days I wouldn't have been out there, but I knew I had to show up. Plus, you're so nervous about every little thing with your first pregnancy and baby, and it's great to just compare notes to know everything's fine."

Even Long-Distance Support Works

Now Lochen and Lindsay are the beneficiaries of this support system. "Larah has been a wealth of information," says Lochen. "Her best advice is basically, 'You can do it.' Being pregnant is scary when everything that you read is about risks and what not to do. She reminded me that I was a healthy, active person and that my baby would probably be so, too."

"Larah's been very helpful because she's had more than one experience, and each was different," adds Lindsay, who's been plagued with nausea and vomiting that still hadn't completely eased up six months into her pregnancy. "She reiterates that I should just do as much as my body will let me, and helps me not freak out. There are so many new things and feelings happening, and I always check in with Larah or Lochen first to make sure what I'm feeling is normal."

Though Lochen was active before she got pregnant, she found new motivation to get in shape when she learned she was expecting. "I wanted to be healthy for my child," she explains. "There's someone inside relying on my health, and that's motivated me the most." She's done some yoga and swimming, but walking and hiking the nearby trails have been her primary exercise. On days when a longer walk isn't an option, she gets in 40 minutes by walking to work, back and forth for lunch, and home again. On weekends, she walks on trails in the subalpine mountains or desert sage. "My pace has just started to slow in the last week or two, now that I'm at 33 weeks. Mostly, my body is just awkward and my breathing is more labored now that the baby takes up more space," she says. "There is one long hill on the Rifle Arch trail that I usually clear without stopping, but the last two times, I've had to stop and catch my breath and let my heart rate slow down." But she wasn't quitting—just adjusting to the changes.

You Can Be Your Pregnant-Best

Exercise has helped Lochen feel physically better, kept her weight gain in check, and more. "Mentally, it's as simple as having that break. And I know walking makes me feel better, because if I skip a few days, my back gets very sore." And though some pregnant women might expect the opposite, Lochen has lost cellulite and gained muscle tone. "My husband says my legs look thinner and more toned now than before," she adds, no doubt due to the combined calorie demands of exercise and pregnancy.

Lindsay, a third-year law student, was used to doing 45 to 60 minutes of cardio and 30 minutes of strength training before she got pregnant and had to cope with morning sickness (or in her case, all-day sickness). "Initially I was very idealistic that I'd keep it all up. Then the sickness hit, and I figured out pretty quickly that I had to do what I was able to do and not any more." In those early months, 20 minutes was a challenge. Now at six months, she's worked back up to 45- to 60-minute walks at a quick pace, four or five days a week, exploring a rail-trail, nearby park, and rural roads with her yellow Lab. "My goals are to exercise for my baby's health, and to be prepared for labor, and keep weight gain to a minimum," she says.

Lessons from the Three Sisters

■ **Hook up with others to walk.** Find someone ready to move at your pace.

■ **Hook up with others to *talk*.** Sisters, friends, doctors; it's natural to have lots of questions, so don't be shy.

■ **Don't have fixed expectations.** You may be able to do more than you thought, or it may be less. Either is okay as long as you're moving.

■ **Don't count on getting great legs during pregnancy,** like Lochen. But don't expect to become a physical wreck, either—this can be a wonderful, very fit and healthy time for you.

GOOD QUESTION

What's great to eat during pregnancy?

Pregnant moms indulged us with a survey of some of their strongest cravings. By no means a "preferred nutrition" list, it will give you a sense of what other moms have gone through:

- "First pregnancy: chicken and cheese enchiladas with lots of hot sauce (girl). Second pregnancy: tortillas with ham, hummus, and cheese (boy)."

- "Pregnancy one: Cortland apples. Pregnancy two: watermelon; whole watermelons (August baby). Pregnancy three: navel oranges. Pregnancy four: pomegranates and mangoes."

- "Coffee-flavored milk."

- "Get this: With Sylvie I was a vegetarian—she loves vegetables! With Mitchell I had lots of french fries—the only meat he eats (if you can call it meat) is fast food burgers or chicken nuggets. With Luc I ate very well and healthy—and Luc eats anything we give him." Coincidence? We don't think so . . .

- "For whatever reason, I ate a lot of sweet potatoes. And hot dogs! (Sick.)"

- "Coconut chocolate chip ice cream cones with chocolate jimmies from Wilbur's Ice Cream Shop. (Used Carl and Debby's nine monthly Wilbur's gift certificates—best shower gift ever!)"

- "Chinese food; chicken fried rice, egg rolls in hot mustard, chicken, broccoli, and cashews, all with lots of soy sauce."

Bottom Line: Fruits and vegetables are nutrient-rich and a great pick if you find them palatable, but sometimes you may just crave things that are more salty and savory. Try for balance, and don't panic if you're not perfect; your walking will help burn off a few (but just a few) extra calories now and then. And remember that drinking plenty of water is still one of the best things you can do for your body.

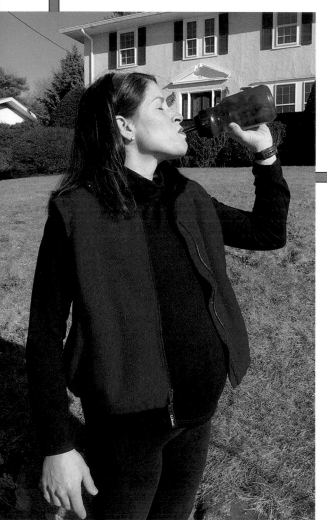

AND FOODS TO STAY AWAY FROM . . .

Elizabeth Ward also offers a reminder of foods to stay away from, to reduce risk of foodborne illness:

- Unheated deli meats.

- Unpasteurized cheeses.

- Raw or undercooked animal foods (sushi, meat, seafood, eggs).

- Avoid fish that may contain excessive mercury: swordfish, shark, king mackerel. Limit shellfish and canned fish to 12 ounces a week; 6 ounces for canned albacore tuna.

When to Back off Exercise

We're pretty adamant in this book that exercise during pregnancy is not just a good idea, but really essential to a healthy, happy pregnancy and quick postpartum recovery. Still, there a few occasions when you may have to back off to make sure you're not putting your baby (or yourself) at risk. Here are some issues to keep an eye on—if you ever have any doubts, you should speak to your doctor immediately.

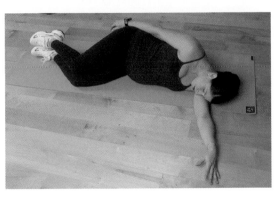

DIASTASIS RECTI—GIVE YOURSELF A QUICK ABDOMINAL CHECK

During pregnancy, women sometimes develop a split or separation in the abdominal (stomach) muscles, called diastasis recti. The abdominal muscles run vertically up the front of your torso, and typically the split occurs right near the middle. It most commonly occurs in the third trimester, or within a few days of delivery, but can happen earlier. It may be the result of the increase of the hormone relaxin, which is softening up ligaments and tissues in anticipation of delivery. But it may also be related to a lack of pre-pregnancy abdominal muscle tone. One study showed that women who are committed to exercise and are fit prior to pregnancy are less likely to develop diastasis—just one more reason to make walking a well-ingrained habit before you conceive.

Do you have Diastasis?

Here's how to check: Lie on your back (or on your left side if you're past the first trimester) with your knees bent. Lift your head off the floor and feel the area in the middle of your stomach, above and below your belly button. If you feel a soft spot in the otherwise firm abdominal wall, or a bulge or ridge pushing through the wall, that indicates diastasis. If you find it, contact your doctor before doing any abdominal exercises. Some specialists believe that continuing to work the torso once you have this separation may make it worse; they recommend you wait until after you deliver to do any strengthening exercises for the abdomen. Others, however, feel there's no danger, so you and your practitioner should decide before you continue abdominal work.

What about after delivery?

Talk to your doctor about how and when it's okay for you to resume abdominal-strengthening exercises. He or she may recommend a supported crunch, where you use a towel as a sling to support your torso. Though strengthening exercises won't heal the split, they will strengthen the other surrounding muscles in the trunk, which are key for maintaining mobility and reducing the likelihood of back pain. If you have trouble finding moves that are comfortable, check with a physical therapist. Remember that it takes time to regain abdominal strength, but by the end of a year you should see considerable improvement. In severe cases, women sometimes opt for surgery to repair the split. If you go this route, it's probably best to wait until you're done having babies.

✳TIP:

Take a natural stride; don't try to force your foot forward to reach for an overly long step. Think about quicker steps—they're the key to faster walking.

A Runner's View of Walking

Elizabeth McGuire, 31, Austin, Texas.

Elizabeth, below, was a competitive runner with five marathons under her belt when she got pregnant. "Staying active came naturally to me because I've been active for a long time and I was already fit," she explains. "I planned to run until it got uncomfortable."

When this began to happen during the sixth month, Elizabeth gradually started to switch from running four to six miles every other day and walking on the off days to all walking. "I walked up the hills or when I got tired. I remember thinking, *I'm running so slowly that I just need to be walking*, plus I was concerned about getting overheated," she recalls. From about seven months, she walked 30 minutes a day, did prenatal yoga once a week, and later swam at least twice a week.

"Walking felt like good exercise and it helped me feel active, not just like I was out there to walk the dog. It was still hard on some days, but it just helped to get out there and move forward."

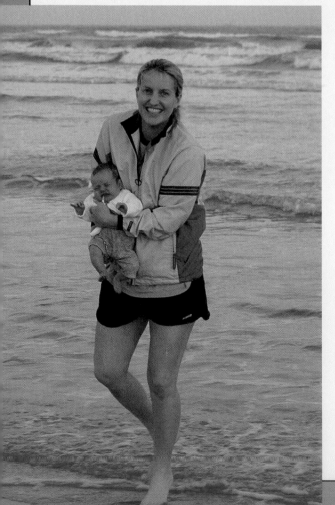

YOU DON'T HAVE TO GIVE UP THE ACTIVE LIFE
Elizabeth's experience offers some lessons for all pregnant women, whether you're a hard-core athlete or just trying to stay active and healthy.

• Swim late in pregnancy. Runners and walkers who miss that fast, light-on-the-feet feeling can get a taste of it in the water, reports Elizabeth. "I never liked swimming but I loved it while I was pregnant. I swam and kicked for about 45 minutes at least twice a week in the last month." *Her tip: Find a quiet pool or at least a quiet time, where you don't have to stress about slowing down speedsters or being out of step with lap etiquette.*

• Use a heart rate monitor. "This was helpful because I was worried about exercising too hard. The monitor set an unwavering limit for me," says Elizabeth. "It was my first pregnancy and I was overly cautious." *Her tip: Use the heart rate monitor for the first few months, until you get a feel for what your pace should be.*

• Seek different types of camaraderie. For part of her pregnancy, Elizabeth ran with a small group of pregnant runners every Saturday. "We compared aches and pains and what we were experiencing," she says. On Wednesday, she ran and then walked with a close friend who matched Elizabeth's pace as her pregnancy progressed. "I would get overwhelmed with the pregnancy chat, so my Wednesday runs were a great balance—we never talked about heartburn or sciatica." *Her tip: Walk with others, but be sure they're ready to walk at your pace.*

- Find a doctor who supports you. "It's similar to wanting a female doctor who has had a baby because you know she's experienced pregnancy firsthand. I knew my doctor already, but if I hadn't I would have chosen her because she's a runner with a child who has been in my shoes. She gave me great guidelines, and she under-stood how fit I was before I got pregnant." *Her tip: Make sure you and your health practitioner talk early and openly about exercise and agree on its importance in a healthy lifestyle.*

THE BEST AND WORST OF IT

The worst part about exercising when pregnant for Elizabeth: "Not knowing how much you can do. Wanting to exercise for yourself, but wondering if that's selfish, and worrying that you might harm the baby."

And the best part: "When you're pregnant, everything is up in the air. You know life is changing, and you don't know what to expect. But exercise is familiar. It's almost like a security blanket."

WHEN DISCRETION IS THE BETTER PART OF VALOR

There are situations in which the risk of aerobic exercise may outweigh the benefits. You need to have a detailed discussion with your doctor describing your desire to remain active and how your walking is feeling. He or she can then decide whether to recommend only specific activities, to limit your exercise intensity or duration, or to advise against exercise altogether based on your particular situation. Here are some of the issues according to the American College of Obstetricians and Gynecologists that may require you to restrict your exercise activity:

- Severe anemia.

- Irregular heart rhythm (in the mother) that has not been evaluated.

- Chronic bronchitis.

- Poorly controlled type 1 diabetes, hypertension, seizure disorder, or hyperthyroidism.

- Extreme obesity or extreme underweight.

- History of extremely sedentary lifestyle.

- Bone, joint, or muscular conditions that cause pain or increase the risk of injury or a fall.

- Habit of smoking heavily (of course, for your health and your baby's you should get help and work to cut down and quit as soon as possible).

 TIP:

Listen to your body—if you're sore, take it easy. If you're fidgety with energy, walk more!

An easy walk can relieve muscle aches and pains, even at very slow speed.

GESTATIONAL DIABETES

Sometime in the second trimester, your doctor will likely give you a glucose tolerance test. You'll be asked to drink several cups of a very sugary (and, by the time you finish, less than appetizing) drink, and then provide a urine sample an hour later. The doctor will be measuring the sugar level in the urine. If it's out of line, it indicates that your body isn't handling the sugar (glucose) properly—you're "glucose intolerant."

This can happen in pregnant moms because of a protective mechanism your body has to ensure that the baby gets enough energy. You normally produce insulin to regulate the amount of glucose in your blood that's being absorbed by your cells for nourishment. Pregnancy triggers processes that keep enough sugar circulating in your bloodstream to nourish your fetus, too. But for some pregnant women the anti-insulin effect is too strong; it keeps excess sugar in the bloodstream, allowing some to pass through the kidneys (which can eventually damage them) and end up in your urine. Most women's bodies balance the mother's and baby's needs, but some simply can't successfully regulate the blood sugar levels. The problem can be temporary, often shows up in the second trimester, and is called gestational diabetes.

GOOD QUESTION

Do any conditions rule out exercise during pregnancy entirely?

Though the medical community is very supportive of women remaining physically active during pregnancy, there are some occasions when a doctor may decide that physical activity—even walking—is simply not a good idea. Following is a list of conditions that would preclude a pregnant woman from doing aerobic exercise, according to the recommendations of the American College of Obstetricians and Gynecologists. It's also possible your doctor may have other concerns not listed here.

- Incompetent cervix. The cervix may open prematurely under the pressure of the growing fetus.
- Ruptured membranes. Leakage of amniotic fluid from the uterus.
- Preeclampsia or pregnancy-induced hypertension. High blood pressure—140/90 or greater—with symptoms including swelling hands and face and rapid weight gain. (Untreated, this can lead to

permanent damage in the mother and growth retardation in the fetus.)

- Placenta previa (after week 26 of the pregnancy). The placenta partially or wholly covers the cervix.
- Bleeding in the second or third trimester that persists.
- Premature labor in this pregnancy.
- Carrying more than one baby where there's a risk for premature labor.
- Some types of heart disease and lung disease.

Bottom Line: You and your doctor have to work closely to determine what's right for your pregnancy. But if you're restricted from exercise, that doesn't mean you've done anything wrong—it simply means that's the best and safest medical course of action for you and your child.

THOSE AT ELEVATED RISK INCLUDE THE FOLLOWING:

- Women with a family history of diabetes.

- Those with a glucose intolerance before pregnancy.

- Overweight and (especially) obese women.

- Women who were large babies themselves or who have had babies over nine pounds.

- Women with obstetrical issues (such as toxemia, repeated urinary tract infections, or excessive amniotic fluid).

- Older women.

Warning signs that you may have gestational diabetes include excessive hunger and thirst, frequent urination even in the second trimester, recurring vaginal infections, and an increase in blood pressure. Though your doctor will routinely give you the test late in the second trimester (sooner if you're at elevated risk), you should speak up if you're feeling these symptoms. Admittedly, many are normal results of pregnancy, so don't panic.

Though this has to be treated and watched carefully, it's really not considered a severe condition. If you're diagnosed with it, your doctor will likely encourage you to exercise—it helps regulate blood sugar levels—and offer strict dietary guidelines. Medication may be necessary, but can ensure a normal pregnancy and healthy baby. And it's reassuring to know that some of the best things you can do to reduce risk are maintain a healthy weight—and keep walking.

TIP:

Get your feet measured every time you buy new shoes. Your feet change over time— especially when you're pregnant— and it's important to buy shoes that fit properly.

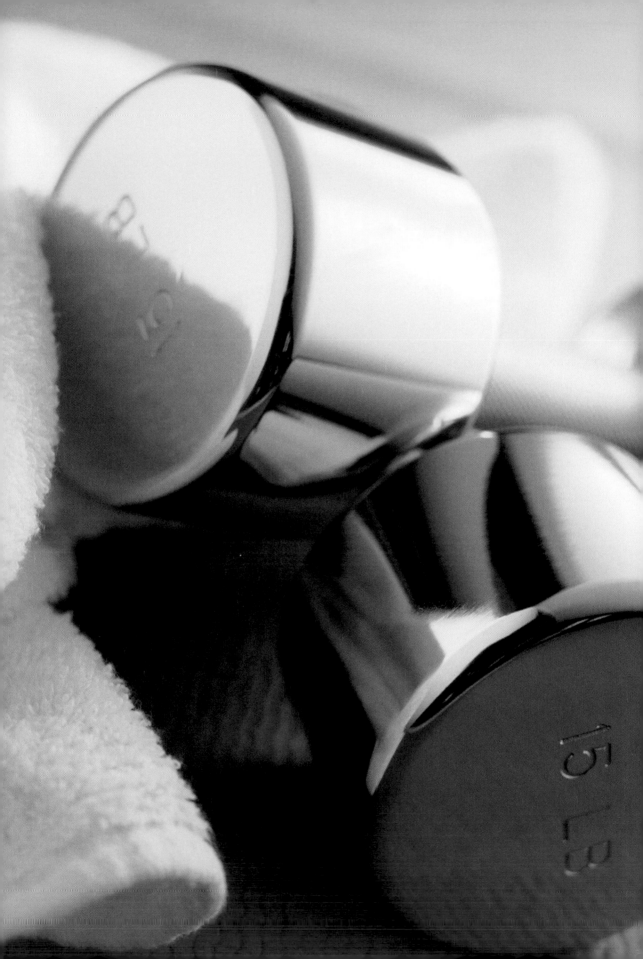

Gear 202: Setting Up for Fitness

Why Take Time to Stretch and Strengthen?

Say the word *exercise* and many women think only of aerobic activities. Step classes, running, swimming, or, our favorite, walking come immediately to mind. But ask the exercise experts, and they'll say that aerobic activity is only one-third of the story, and if that's all you do then you're selling yourself short. In fact, the American College of Sports Medicine recommendations—designed for the public at large but entirely relevant to pregnant women—suggest three specific components for overall fitness:

1. **AEROBIC ACTIVITY.** This is the key to maintaining cardiovascular fitness—the fitness that keeps you from being winded after pulling your growing body up a flight of stairs. It can also burn plenty of calories, helping assure that you put weight on at a healthy, not horrifying, rate. The ACSM likes any activity that causes you to move your big muscles for 20 to 60 minutes, at least three to five days a week. This means that everything from running to bicycling to swimming counts, but it's got to be either very regular (five or more days a week) or pretty intense (enough to get you breathing hard at least three days a week) to really build cardio fitness. A favorite is walking because it's easiest on a pregnant body, and simple to adjust to your fitness level and how you're feeling. A novice can take daily neighborhood strolls; a more experienced athlete can opt for shorter sweat-inducing power walks or longer leg-burning hikes in the hills now and then.

2. **STRENGTH.** This helps keep your posture in line and your body able to carry its added weight while still doing the work of daily life. Any sort of resistance exercise can do the job—calisthenics and floor exercises, using stretchy bands or tubing, lifting dumbbells or larger free weights, or any of the myriad exercise machines you can find in gyms and health clubs. Eventually even (for *some* moves) gently and carefully lifting your new child can build strength. The key is to exercise all the major muscle groups (six to eight exercises can cover most of the arms and shoulders, trunk, and legs) two or more days per week. The experts suggest doing at least two sets of each exercise, with from 8 to 12 repetitions (lifts) in each set.

3. **FLEXIBILITY.** Again, you can choose the activity—static stretching moves, yoga—but the goal is to devote at least a few minutes every day to maintaining a healthy range of movement in your joints. Don't stress about trying to become as flexible as a world-class

gymnast. It takes a ton of time, and for average folks the benefits aren't clear. You just want to do enough to make sure your tissues don't tighten up so much that you can't grab the bulk groceries off the top shelf, or do the extreme reach for the sippy cup rolling around under the backseat of the car. In other words, at least keep the mobility you have now and steer clear of future injury.

The upshot of this is that building at least a little stretching and strengthening into your routine is just as important as walking. In fact, a regular, moderate stretching and strengthening routine not only helps keep you looking and feeling better, but also assures you don't risk injury from such mundane moves as opening a stiff window or lifting your pregnant body up and down the stairs—an issue now—or lifting the baby in or out of a car seat or high chair—an issue sooner than you might think!

Stretch-and-Strengthen Hardware

Stretching and strengthening is easier and more likely to happen if you've got some basic equipment at home. You only need a few items, and then you're ready whenever you get a spare 15 minutes. No gym membership or commute required.

There's a wide range of gear on the market to help you build strength, but for the sake of simplicity, we recommend the basics. The pieces described below are all-around winners: versatile, effective, simple to use, easy to store, and inexpensive.

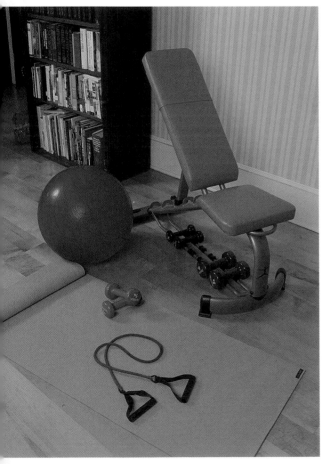

FLOOR MATS

Thin, foam mats are an inexpensive way to make the floor a cushy, safe surface for working out. If you've got hardwood floors (ouch) or area rugs (yikes, slippery), a floor mat provides a thin, nonslip surface that won't interfere as you stretch or strengthen. If you have a room with wall-to-wall carpet that's not too plush or slippery, you can probably get away without a mat; even then, however, the mat gets you away from what can be a scratchy, irritating surface. Mats come in a variety of sizes; look for one that's 20 to 24 inches by 48 to 56 inches so your moves aren't cramped.

COST: $13–$60.

UPSIDE: The comfort can make the difference between getting motivated to do that toning or yoga session, and skipping it altogether.

DOWNSIDE: One more thing to store.

LOOK FOR: A mat with a grippy or textured non-slip surface (bare feet and sweaty skin won't lose grip); easy rolling or folding for compact storage.

NICE EXTRAS: Some are sanitized to prevent bacteria and fungi from setting up camp.

BRANDS INCLUDE: Airex, AeroMAT, Reebok, SPRI.

A Simple Home Gym

Allison and John Librett, Atlanta, Georgia

Allison and John Librett, below with Sophie, have both been dedicated to active living, so it's no surprise they've kept it up even since the birth of children Sophie (3) and Nicholas (1). One key to their success has been setting up a home gym. It's nothing fancy, but Allison says it's been a lifesaver when getting out the door simply isn't an option.

THEIR KEY PIECES ARE:

- Dumbbells in 5-, 10-, 15-, and 20-pound increments.
- Medicine ball (if you're not sure, start with five to eight pounds).
- Elastic exercise bands.
- Yoga mat.
- Bike stand.

The last one converts Allison's bicycle to a stationary bike right on the porch, allowing her to jump on whenever a chunk of time materializes. The full setup assures that in a pinch she can get in all the components of fitness—aerobics (a bike ride), flexibility, and strength—without leaving home.

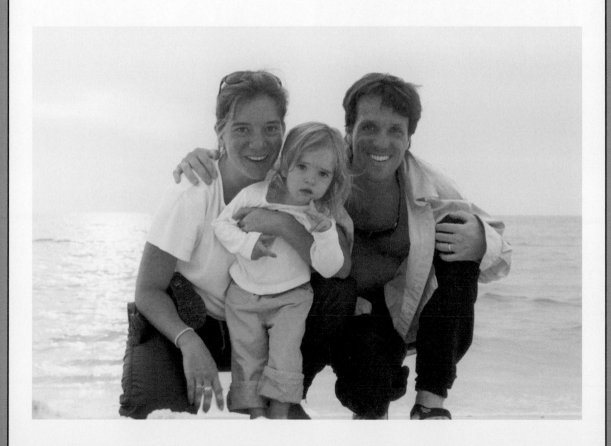

DUMBBELLS

Smart equipment for basic strength building, dumbbells can be used to work the upper body through a wide variety of patterns and moves. Dumbbells are sold in pairs or sometimes by the pound. You can buy the traditional cast-iron types (like the ones in your high school gym) or flashier coated or rubberized versions that cost a bit more.

Cost: Roughly $.50 per pound for basic iron; about $1.20 per pound for shiny chrome, and $5–$25 a pair for vinyl covered, depending on weight increment.

Upside: Simple to use, and effective for all sorts of upper-body moves.

Downside: As you get stronger, you may need another heavier pair.

Look for: Neoprene- or vinyl-covered weights are more comfortable to hold than plain old iron. If you've never lifted weights, get pairs of 2-, 3-, and 5-pound dumbbells. If you're fit or you've

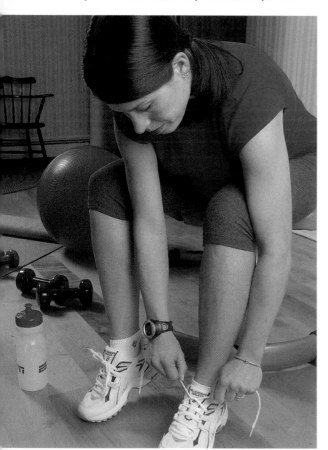

been weight training at a gym, go with 5- and 8- or 10-pounders. You may think you want more, but start conservatively—you don't want to push too hard at first, and can always buy another pair if you turn out to be superwoman.

Where to find them: Locally, sporting goods or big-box stores (Wal-Mart, Sears, and the like) often have sets such as 2-, 3-, and 5-pounders for $25–$35. Online, try sites such as Perform Better, SPRI, and MegaFitness.

RESISTANCE BANDS OR TUBING

If dumbbells seem cumbersome, burly, or too tough to store, opt for stretchy bands of elasticized tubing with handles attached to both ends. The color-coded bands come in different tensions. Get two or three for a variety of moves, and so you can make your workout more challenging as you get stronger, or easier if your energy flags late in pregnancy.

Cost: $5–$25 per band. More expensive bands are more durable and may come with a warranty and sample exercises.

Upside: Less bulk than dumbbells. Packable and portable. Can be used to strengthen both the upper and the lower body.

Downside: It takes some experimenting to find the band that delivers the right amount of tension, and a bit of practice to learn to move smoothly.

Look for: Color-coding so you can easily grab the right tension; comfortable handle grips, large enough to slip your foot through for moves when you pull against your feet.

Nice extras: A door anchor allows you to attach the tubing to a fixed position for more variety.

Brands include: Xertube, Lifeline, Stretch Cordz, J.C.

Where to find them: Locally at sporting goods or big-box stores; by phone or online at sites such as SPRI, Perform Better, and MegaFitness.

FITNESS BALLS

They look like they belong at a kid's fun house, but these oversized inflatable balls do serious work. Also known as Swiss balls, stability balls, and balance balls, they're great for all kinds of stretching

GOOD QUESTION

Why is it so important to drink a lot of water?

You constantly hear that you're supposed to drink at least eight 8-ounce glasses of water a day. And no doubt you've been warned that for an exercising pregnant woman, staying well hydrated is especially important. That's because during exercise, your rate of fluid loss (and the risk of overheating) can be especially high. Here's why you want to make sure you keep the fluid tank comfortably full:

- Water aids in the digestion and absorption of foods through the intestinal walls.

- Water is critical in the elimination of metabolic wastes.

- Your body's thermoregulatory system depends heavily on water. If you don't have enough water to sweat, you can't receive the natural cooling benefit of water evaporating on your skin.

- The majority of your blood is water, so being well hydrated is central to maintaining a healthy blood volume. One way you dissipate extra heat is by sending blood to your skin's surface so that excess heat can escape—it's why you look flushed and your skin is warm to the touch. But if your blood volume drops, this cooling process is impaired. You can also experience an unnaturally elevated heart rate and drop in blood pressure—both especially unhealthy for a pregnant woman and her baby.

- Water can be a healthy and natural appetite suppressant. Certainly drinking water frequently can help give a sense of fullness. But you may find that there are times when you're tempted to eat something cold and savory (say, ice cream) when in fact you're really quite thirsty. A cold glass of water might actually be the better choice. (Which is not to say you should ignore a craving for calcium—just watch out for that tag-along fat!)

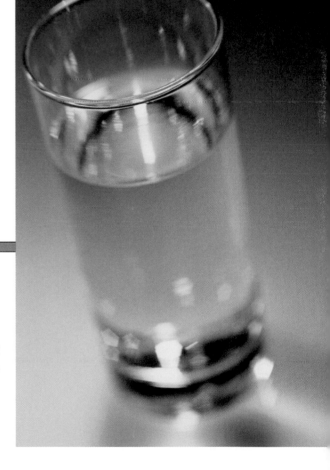

and strengthening moves, with or without dumbbells. (Many hospitals have them in their labor units because some laboring women find them comfortable to stretch or rest on.) Fitness balls come in different sizes; the taller you are, the bigger the ball you need. A good rule of thumb: Make sure when you sit on the ball, your thighs are parallel to the floor. If you're five feet tall to five-seven, go with a 55-centimeter ball. If you're from five-eight to six-three, you need a 65-centimeter ball.
Cost: $20–$30, plus $13–$25 for a pump.
Upside: Fun to use. Great for building balance and stability.
Downside: It takes a little time to learn what to do with them. Bulky.
Look for: An antiburst ball. If it gets punctured, it deflates slowly, so you won't crash to the floor.
Brands include: Gymnic, Resist-A-Ball, FlexaBall.
Where to find them: Local sporting goods or big-box stores; online or by telephone: Ball Dynamics, OPTP, Perform Better, SPRI.

Beat the heat
with morning
or evening
walks. Drink
early and
often during
warm-
weather
walks.

Water, Water Everywhere—
Have You Enough to Drink?

Since staying well hydrated is important when you're pregnant, and even more so when you're active or exercising, you may have to think about how to bring water along on walks. For short outings (under 30 to 45 minutes) and in cool weather, it's enough to just drink before and after your walk. But for longer workouts or in hot or humid conditions, you'll need to carry fluids. That's where the proper gear comes in. Your options range from a simple reusable plastic water bottle from the supermarket to a technical backpack equipped with a water pouch.

BASIC WATER BOTTLES

With a flip top for easy and fast filling and cleaning, these plastic water bottles are cheap, reusable, and very handy. You can stow water bottles in a range of waist packs and belts with loops and holders designed specifically to hold bottles; the problem is that with your expanding belly, that's only good for the first few months of pregnancy at most.

Upside: Inexpensive, at $2-$10; you won't fret if you lose one. Carrying the cold bottle can even help you feel a bit cooler.

Downside: You have to carry them by hand, or if you stow them in a knapsack you have to stop to take them in and out when you need a drink. Can be awkward on long walks or in hot weather, when you'll need to carry more water.

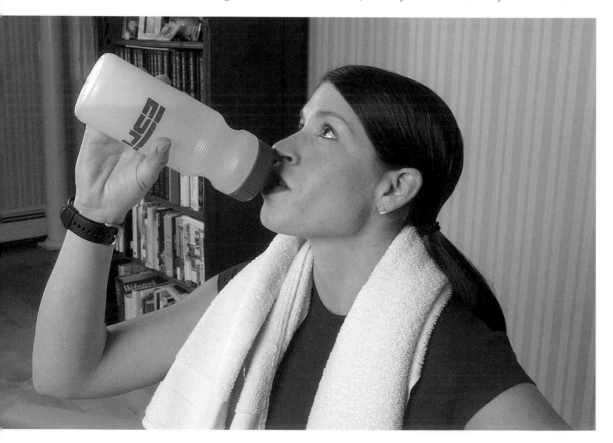

Look for: A wide mouth for popping in ice cubes; 12 to 16 ounces of capacity—more will be cumbersome to carry.

Nice extras: Grippy sides, contours, or hand straps for easy carrying. Insulation to keep contents cold.

Where to find them: Local grocery stores, sporting goods stores, bike and running specialty shops.

WATER BLADDER OR RESERVOIR

This plastic pouch can be filled with lots of water (usually one or two liters) and set inside your backpack. A long tube with a mouth valve runs back to the pouch in your pack, so you can drink whenever you want. (Some packs come with a "port" or opening for the tube to pass through at the top of the pack. Otherwise, you have to snake it out through the zipper or flap.)

Cost: About $25 and up.

Upside: Comfortable way to carry lots of water. Great for longer outings and hot weather. With the tube near at hand, you may be inclined to sip more regularly.

Downside: Can be awkward to clean and refill.

Look for: A soft mouthpiece that's comfortable in your mouth; a wide opening for ice cubes.

Brands include: CamelBak, Kelty, Platypus.

HYDRATION SYSTEMS AND HYDRATION-EQUIPPED BACKPACKS

Don't be intimidated by the technical names. These are simply water carriers that you wear backpack style, or backpacks that come already loaded with a water reservoir, tube, and mouthpiece. Though you can also find waist packs with similar setups, save those for after the baby is born. Given your growing belly, you'll be much better off with a backpack style now.

Upside: The most comfortable and convenient way to carry and drink on a long walks or day hikes. Most hold two liters of water plus have easy-access compartments for stowing the rest of your food, gear, and clothing.

Downside: Pricey. A minimal pack that holds two liters starts at about $60.

Look for: A soft mouthpiece; a wide opening for adding ice cubes; comfortable and adjustable padded shoulder straps with a clip to hold the water tube, to keep it accessible and not flopping around; easy access to gear stashed in the pack.

Nice extras: Some companies make models specifically to fit a women's torso.

Brands include: CamelBak, Kelty, L.L. Bean.

Where to find them: Look at hiking stores and outdoor outfitters such as REI, L.L. Bean, and EMS.

TIP:

At the end of your walk, stroll slowly and give your body a few minutes to cool down. This allows your muscles to relax gently, lets your heart rate lower gradually, and prevents blood from pooling in your legs.

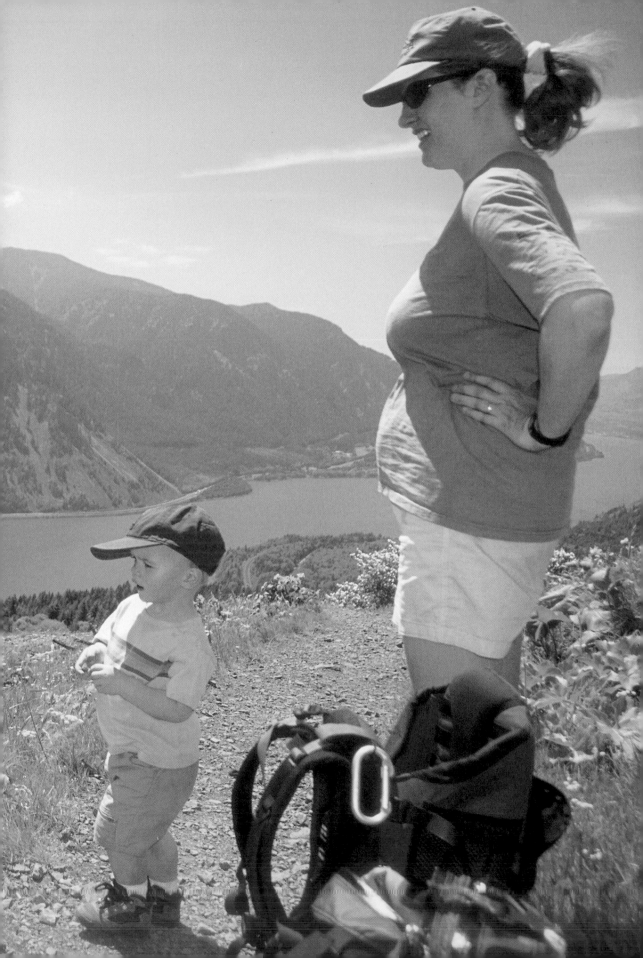

The Walking Program, Trimester II

Am I Walking Fast Enough (or Too Fast)?

The increased energy you're likely feeling in the second trimester may also have you thinking about whether you're really exercising hard enough. Your weight gain is likely a bit more noticeable, and you may be concerned that you're getting too much too soon, with your fitness dropping off too rapidly. But the weight gain is normal and healthy, and if you're feeling good and have the doctor's okay, this is actually the ideal time to gradually increase the intensity and duration of your exercise. A perfect way to do this is to pick up the pace of your walks on one or two days of the week, and make your walks a bit longer on another day or two. Measuring increases in walking duration is easy—just keep an eye on your watch, and add a few minutes to your longest walk every week or so. But boosting speed is trickier. Unless you walk around a track or on a treadmill, it's hard to gauge how fast you're going. Still, it turns out there's a simple way to know if you're really giving your walk a boost.

COUNT STEPS FOR YOUR SPEED

Not surprisingly, the faster you walk, the more steps you have to take in a minute. What *is* surprising is that the relationship is pretty predictable, meaning your step rate actually provides a very simple way to estimate your walking speed. It's not as accurate as timing yourself on a track, but it will give a decent estimate you can use to compare yourself from one walk to the next. Want to see if you're getting more fit and walking faster? Count your steps at two or three points during your walk. If you're averaging a higher step rate than previous workouts, you can be sure that you're actually walking faster. Counting your steps now and then has another advantage: It makes you more conscious of your effort, and that alone may help make your walk a better workout.

Here's how to estimate your walking speed: After you're warmed up during a walk, glance at your watch and count how many steps you take in a minute. You can count for a full 60 seconds, or you can just count for 20 seconds and multiply by three. (If you're walking especially fast, it may be easier to count only when your right or left foot hits the ground and double that answer.) You now have your step rate, in steps/minute. Find that figure under the appropriate column for your height in the "Step Rate Table," and follow it to the right to estimate your walking speed.

STEP RATE TABLE *Estimate speed based on steps in a minute.*				
STEP RATE (STEPS/MINUTE)			WALKING SPEED (MPH)	TIME TO WALK 1 MILE (MIN:SEC)
Height < 5'6"	Height 5'6"–6'	Height > 6'		
100–110	95–105	90–100	2.0	30:00
105–115	100–110	95–105	2.5	24:00
110–120	105–115	100–110	3.0	20:00
120–130	115–125	110–120	3.5	17:10
130–140	125–135	120–130	4.0	15:00
140–150	135–145	130–140	4.5	13:20
155–165	150–160	145–155	5.0	12:00

GOOD QUESTION

How do I maintain healthy walking technique?

Though increasing weight and a shifting center of mass may make it seem unlikely, it's more important than ever to try to walk with a tall, healthy posture. It will help reduce stiffness and keep your body aligned. Three things in particular will help you maintain a healthy gait:

- **Eyes on the horizon.** Stand tall and keep your gaze forward, not down at the ground in front of you. This will help keep your head up and shoulders back, not slouched forward.

- **Tuck your butt underneath.** Excuse the bluntness, but if you feel you're pulling your buttocks underneath you (by tilting the top of your pelvis back, not forward), it will help reduce excess arch in your lower back.

- **Don't overstride.** There's no need to reach forward with your heel, and doing so can strain your hamstrings (back of the thigh) and gluteal muscles. Just take a natural-feeling step.

Good technique is especially helpful as you pick up the pace:

- **Take quicker steps.** Focus on taking faster rather than longer steps; your stride will lengthen as your pace quickens, but don't force it.

- **Roll off your toes.** Imagine showing someone behind you the sole of your sneaker at the end of every step, by pushing off your toes.

- **Bend your arms.** Not only do you get a bit more of an upper-body workout, but you'll walk faster if you bend your arms 90 degrees at the elbow. Your hands should trace an arc from next to the waistband on the backswing, to letter height on a T-shirt (and no higher) in front with this quick, compact arm swing.

Bottom Line: Healthy walking technique depends on good tall posture and a natural stride, with eyes looking forward not down, shoulders back, chest open, and lower back as flat as is reasonable. To pick up the pace, focus on quicker rather than longer strides, bend your arms, and push off your toes at the end of each stride.

GOOD QUESTION

Is it true that a taller person can walk faster than a shorter one simply because of her longer legs?

In a word, no. So if you're in a walking group with other pregnant women, and a shorter one is complaining about the pace, the issue is not height. It may be that some folks are more or less fit, or are heavier, or interested in a harder workout. But it's unlikely height is the reason. Here's why:

Your walking speed depends on two things: the length of your stride, and the speed of your steps. You can speed up by taking longer steps, or by taking more steps each minute, or a combination. A taller person has an advantage when it comes to taking longer steps—longer legs simply mean she has a longer natural stride.

But who has the advantage when it comes to taking faster steps? The shorter person. That's because someone with shorter legs has less of a pendulum (that's all the leg is, really) to swing forward on each step, and she has to put less energy into it. This means the short-legged person can take faster steps with less effort.

So who's got the leg up, as it were? Is it better for long strides to come naturally, or for fast strides to be effortless? In fact, the short person may be better off! You can only increase the length of your stride a certain amount, then it would become absurd—right out of Monty Python's Ministry of Silly Walks. But there's not such a clear limit to stride rate—as you become fitter and fitter, you can make your steps faster and faster. In fact, competitive racewalkers holding speeds over 8 mph maintain well over 200 steps per minute for 12 miles! Which is one reason that shorter people are often very successful at the highest levels of competition. America's top-ranked female racewalker for many years was a women less than five feet, three inches tall (and a mother of three, to boot).

Bottom Line: Tall walkers take longer strides, but shorter walkers can take faster strides with less effort, and these are largely balancing effects. So if two people of different heights can't walk together, it's probably because one is more fit or working harder, not because of the height difference.

HOW FAST IS FAST?

Consider 2.0 to 2.5 mph a window-shopping pace for most women. About 3.0 to 3.5 mph is a typical healthy walking pace—if done regularly, it's enough to provide reduced risk for chronic disease, and it's a great target for novice exercisers and those really starting to feel their pregnancy weight. Push into the 3.5 to 4.0 mph range and you'll boost the cardio benefits measurably. Most women will be boosting the effort, too—a challenging but still-comfortable fitness walking tempo. For most people, 4.5 mph and above is a true power walking pace—they have to very consciously think about quickening their steps and bending their arms to get into this highly aerobic range. Unless you're a fit and experienced walker, don't expect (or try) to sustain these speeds for more than 10 to 20 minutes in a workout.

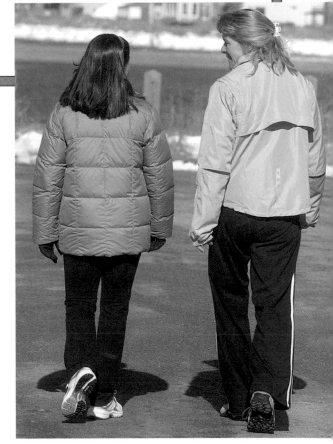

TIP:

Well-cushioned, synthetic socks are worth the price. Avoid cotton clothing in cold, wet weather.

As you progress into the third trimester, however, be prepared to see all of those speeds reduced by at least 0.5 mph, and even more as you approach delivery. So as you get into your ninth month, don't be surprised or depressed if it feels like your pace has dropped off by as much as one mile per hour or more. That's not a sign that you're falling apart, but simply a result of all the extra weight you're carrying out front.

Is It Time to Hit the Weights?

It's easy to understand why walking is the ideal aerobic activity during pregnancy. It's a simple, inexpensive, natural low-impact activity that everyone knows how to do, and can maintain right up to delivery. But how big a place does resistance (or strength) training have in the pregnancy exercise mix? We're talking about anything from lifting free weights or using resistance machines to doing floor exercises or working with stretchy bands. In fact, it provides benefits that walking simply can't. Here are the most notable:

▪ Resistance training really helps you maintain lean body mass (that is, muscle). That's critical for holding to a healthy rate of weight gain during pregnancy, because muscle is your body's best calorie burner.

GOOD QUESTION

Do I put my baby at risk by lifting weights while pregnant?

No, as long as your pregnancy is progressing normally, resistance exercise isn't a problem. It's actually a good idea to help maintain muscle tone and strength, and you'll probably find that it helps you maintain healthier posture and alleviate some of the strain that comes with carrying extra baby weight. But it is important to use good technique, never stress yourself, and follow these guidelines when strength training:

▪ Concentrate on good, slow technique—don't let momentum do the work for you—and move your joints through their full range of motion.

▪ Exhale while lifting the weight; inhale on the recovery or between reps.

▪ Maintain good posture. Focus on stabilizing your body throughout all movements, especially with your abdominal and back muscles. If you can't, then you're lifting too much weight.

▪ Pick a weight so that you can do an exercise 8 to 10 times in a row (that's one set of 8 to 10 repeti-

tions); then rest briefly and do another set of 8 to 10 repetitions. Then move to the next exercise.

▪ Lifting shouldn't hurt, but it should be challenging. Select a weight (or loop your resistance band or stretch tubing) so that you're feeling muscle fatigue on the last repetitions of each set of each exercise. But never be straining or grunting to finish.

▪ Do exercises in the order shown, beginning with larger muscle groups, and working toward smaller ones. Always exercise both parts of a muscle pair (say, both the muscles that both extend a joint, and those that flex it).

▪ Keep progressing. When a weight becomes easy to lift, add more. Increase to the next weight and reduce the number of repetitions, if necessary, until you're able to build up to the full target number again.

- You need strength in daily life. Even as your body changes during pregnancy, you'll remain stronger and better prepared for everyday tasks, as well as a few new ones. (After all, who'll be carrying the baby every day? And painting his room, too?)

- Your body will remain a little more familiar. No doubt with pregnancy your belly will bulge, breasts will grow, and posture will shift. But the more toned your muscles, the more you'll maintain a lean look and defined feel. You may be changing, but that doesn't mean you have to feel like a soft, droopy slug.

- Specific exercises can help stave off pregnancy-related problems. Reducing low-back pain and preventing ankle swelling and varicose veins can be aided by proper strength-training moves.

- It's probably an advantage during delivery. Though no research establishes that fitter women have shorter labor, many women indicate that feeling fit and strong going in helped them cope with the physical challenge they faced.

- You'll come back faster after delivery. Keep muscles stronger now, and you're guaranteed to regain your pre-pregnancy form even faster after delivery.

If you've been doing strength training of some sort and you want to keep going during pregnancy, you certainly should with your doctor's okay. Most women will find their doctors very encouraging, given all the benefits just mentioned. But now is not the time to try to bump up your weight totals or add challenging new exercises. Instead, modify your routine and choose weights that minimize strain, eliminate discomfort, and assure you can maintain healthy posture throughout the movements. Most important, replace exercises where you lie on your back with alternative moves lying on your side, sitting, or standing up.

If you don't have a recent history of resistance training, fear not. There are lots of options, from free weights and resistance machines to floor exercises and stretch bands (see chapter 5), to combination strength and stretching activities, such as yoga and Pilates. If you've tried and enjoyed one of those in the past, keep it up or go back to it, keeping in mind the warnings below. But if you haven't got a favorite activity, the simple strength routine outlined below is a good place to start.

SIMPLE STRENGTH ROUTINE

This routine is designed so you can do it in a minimally equipped gym or even at home. Ideally you'll have some stretch bands or small dumbbells (3 to 10 pounds), a bench or sturdy chair, and a floor mat—all easy to find. The one odd bit of hardware is an open door for the lat pulls. It's great to have a wall mirror, too, so you can keep an eye on your form and in particular your posture. You want to remain tall and keep your trunk stable through all the moves.

TIP:
Wear bright reflective colors if you're walking in the dark, or even at dawn or dusk. Never walk down dark alleys alone. Never walk very fast with scissors in your hands.

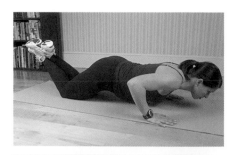

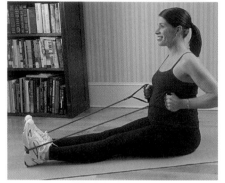

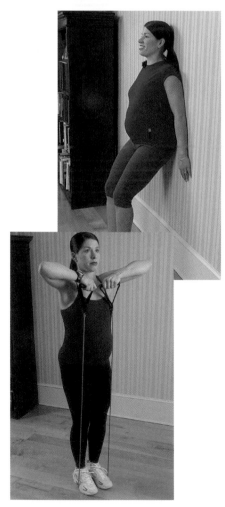

1 **Knee push-ups.** (For chest, shoulders, arms, overall strength; supports breasts.) Begin on your hands and knees, with your hands shoulder width apart. Bend your arms and lower your chest to the floor, keeping your back as straight as possible. Then push back up to the start position. Try for 10 repetitions (one set); rest, then try for 10 more. *If too easy:* Push your hands farther forward, away from your knees, but not so much that you feel discomfort or a noticeable sway in your lower back while doing them. If you're very strong you may even be able to do full push-ups for a while, supporting yourself on just your toes and hands. Do these only as long as you can keep your legs and torso straight throughout the push-up. *If too hard:* Place your hands and knees closer together, and don't go down so low. Or do wall push-ups: Stand just under arm's length from a wall, placing your hands on the wall just below shoulder height. Bend your elbows and lean into the wall from your ankles, then push away to stand upright.

2 **Seated rowing.** (For back, shoulders, arms, overall strength; improves posture.) Sit with your legs straight out in front of you, back straight and tall. Loop a resistance band around or over your feet. Pull straight back with both hands, pulling the band toward your chest and elbows back, so that you squeeze your shoulder blades together at the end of the pull, then slowly return to start. Do 10 repetitions; rest, then do 10 more. *If too easy:* Choose a higher-tension band, or loop it farther away on a table leg. Or try bent-over rows with dumbbells (see the program in chapter 18). *If too hard:* Use a band with lower tension, or even one band for each foot/hand.

3 **Pelvic tilt.** (For abdominal muscles; reduces excess arch in the lower back.) Stand with your feet about eight inches from a wall, shoulder width apart. With knees slightly bent, place your back against the wall, keeping your knees above your feet (no farther forward). Gently contract your stomach muscles, attempting to tilt your pelvis back (you should feel you're tucking your butt under you) and flatten your lower back against the wall. Hold for three slow, deep breaths (about 10 seconds) then release. Do five repetitions; rest, then do five more. *If too easy:* Move your feet closer to the wall, and increase to eight repetitions. *If too hard:* Move your feet farther from the wall; if needed, only hold for five seconds until you're stronger. **Alternative:** This may be easier or more comfortable. Begin on your hands and knees, with your back flat (not sagging downward). Gently contract your abdominal muscles and curve your back upward, then slowly relax to the back-flat position. Do 10 slow repetitions; relax, then repeat with another set of 10.

4 **Upright row.** (For upper shoulders, arms, and those soon-to-be-needed baby-lifting muscles.) Stand with your feet shoulder width apart, arms extended downward, palms facing back, hands holding stretch bands looped under your feet. Keeping your elbows high, pull your hands up to in front of your shoulders, then return to start. Do 10 repetitions; rest, then do 10 more. *If too easy:* Choose a higher-tension band. Or do these with dumbbells. *If too hard:* Use a band with lower tension, or even one band for each foot/hand.

5 Lat pull-downs. (For the arms; for the muscles—latissimus dorsi—along the sides of the back; for posture and core strength.) Sit at the front of a chair facing the edge of an open door, with your legs straddling the door and arms extended upward grasping a stretch band looped over the door. Pull your arms down to shoulder height, then return to start. Do 10 repetitions; rest, then do 10 more. *If too easy:* Choose a higher-tension band or a lat pull-down machine at a gym. Very strong women may (for a while) be able to do pull-ups on an overhead bar (begin with a helper to spot you until you're more experienced). *If too hard:* Use a band with lower tension; stand, to reduce the length of the pull.

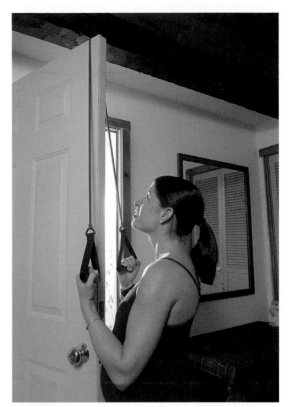

6 Abdominal oblique crunch. (For side of the abdominal muscles; aids posture and trunk strength.) Lie on your left side with your knees slightly bent, your shoulders, hips, and ankles in a line, and your left arm extended on the floor in front of you. Reach for your feet with your right hand, trying to lift your upper body slightly off the ground (you may push a bit with your left hand to help); you don't have to lift high at all to feel the muscles on the side of the abdomen working. Do eight repetitions, then switch sides and repeat. Then do another set on each side. *If too easy:* Don't push up at all with your hand on the ground; try for 10, 12, or 15 repetitions per set. *If too hard:* Don't try to lift so high; start with five repetitions per set.

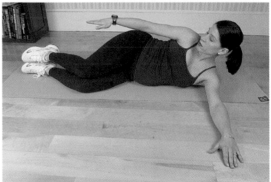

7 Biceps curl. (For the front of the upper arm—another baby-lifting muscle.) Stand with your feet shoulder width apart, arms extended downward, hands facing palm forward, holding stretch bands looped under your feet. Keeping your elbows tucked in close to your body, bend your arms and pull your hands up to in front of your shoulders, then return to start. Do 10 repetitions; rest, then do 10 more. *If too easy:* Choose a higher-tension band. Or do biceps curls with dumbbells (see program in chapter 18). *If too hard:* Use a band with lower tension, or one band for each foot/hand.

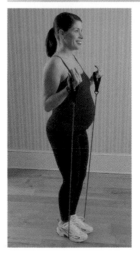

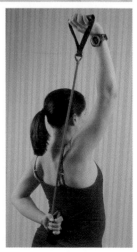

8 Triceps extension. (For back of the upper arm; for pushing and lifting.) Stand with your feet shoulder width apart, holding the stretch band behind your back in one hand, with your other arm overhead, bent at the elbow, holding the other end. Keeping your lower arm still, pressed against your back, extend the overhead arm straight up in the air, then return to start. Do 10 repetitions; rest, then do 10 more. *If too easy:* Choose a higher-tension band. Or do triceps extensions with dumbbells (see program in chapter 18). *If too hard:* Use a band with lower tension.

GOOD QUESTION

Why does the walking program always show at least one day off a week?

The simple answer is that in a normal busy life, it's not uncommon to have at least one day a week when things are so chaotic—you have nonstop meetings, your sitter is sick—that you simply can't get in a walk. Call that your day off, be active the rest of the week, and you'll be right on target with the program.

But a sports physiologist's answer is that when exercising regularly, your body needs a break to keep improving in fitness. Improving or maintaining fitness is a "stress response." You stress your heart and muscles during exercise—making the heart beat at an accelerated rate, say, or forcing muscles to lift heavier-than-usual loads—and they respond by trying to build themselves up in response to the challenge.

But your tissues actually need time to repair and even strengthen themselves, especially after hard exercise. Add in the physiological demands of pregnancy, and rest becomes an even more urgent need. That's why the program suggests alternating longer and shorter walks, it spreads faster walks over the week (not back to back), and it suggests taking the day off after the longest walk each week. These variations all combine to give the body a chance to recover, and to rebuild more successfully.

Bottom Line: For fitness to be maintained or improve, the body needs time to rebuild, especially after hard exercise. So the more challenging workouts (longer or faster walks) are interspersed with shorter, easier recovery walks, and at least one day a week off from exercise entirely. This variety is especially important for pregnant women because of the additional demands of pregnancy on your body.

The Second-Trimester Walking Program

GENERAL REMINDERS FOR TRIMESTER II

▪ Keep listening to your body. Your body is strong and conditions are fairly stable, so if you're feeling good now is the time to gently boost the length and even intensity of some of your walks.

▪ But make the increases gradually. You don't want to shock your system. Take note of your weekly mileage or walking time (using your training log) and the speed of your walks (say, using the step-counting method), and don't increase either by more than 5 to 10 percent from one week to the next.

▪ As always, if anything feels wrong or discomfort persists, back off and check with your doctor.

▪ Still use short walks, too. On days you're tired or don't feel good, don't be lulled into thinking that blowing off your walk is the right call. Sometimes a short walk (or two) can actually help. Get out the door just for five minutes, and see where it leads.

▪ Maintain muscle tone. The easy warm-ups and after-walk stretch routines not only promote healthy joints and tissues, but even provide a bit of resistance exercise.

▪ Make strength training a part of your routine, from two to four days a week, depending on what you've done before.

▪ Do Kegels daily. The medical community recommends doing sets of 10 contraction exercises (hold for several seconds and relax) two or three times a day. Master these simple isometric exercises, and fit them in every day.

LOW-KEY PROGRAM, TRIMESTER II

By now you should be homing in on what it takes to get out and walk five days a week. Your doctor swears your nausea is subsiding and your energy level is returning, which makes this trimester the ideal time to build up to six days of walking a week. You can also modestly increase your total walking time, at least on the days you're feeling the best. Continue to work on a daily stretching habit, doing the quick stretch routine after most walks. If you've had success with the quick stretches, then it's time to start doing the full stretch routine (shown in chapter 3) whenever you can. You'll gain the added benefit of better flexibility maintenance plus some muscle toning with this more full-body series of moves.

GOALS FOR A TYPICAL WEEK

▪ Continue walking at least five days a week, but begin adding another day whenever possible, to average six days of walking a week by midtrimester. It's still okay if some of those are just 10- to 15-minute walks.

▪ Slowly add walking minutes. Gradually over the weeks add a few minutes of walking, every several days. By week 22, try to average two 25- to 30-minute walks and three or four 15- to 20-minute walks per week.

▪ Continue to break your walks up if it helps.

▪ Do the simple warm-ups before, and quick stretch routine after, as many walks as possible. (Both shown in chapter 3.)

A TYPICAL WEEK IN MID-TO LATE TRIMESTER II, LOW-KEY PROGRAM:							
	MON.	TUES.	WED.	THUR.	FRI.	SAT.	SUN.
WALK (minutes)	25	20	25	15	10, 10	30	OFF
OTHER STUFF	WARM-UPS, FULL FLEX	WARM-UPS, FULL FLEX	WARM-UPS, QUICK STRETCH	WARM-UPS	WARM-UPS, QUICK STRETCH	WARM-UPS, FULL FLEX	

MODERATE PROGRAM, TRIMESTER II

If you had a history of at least somewhat regular exercise before pregnancy, and you now have three months of experience with your changing body, now is the perfect time for you to really get back into the groove. You should firmly establish the habit of six days of exercise per week, with proper warm-ups and stretches. Now is the time to slowly increase the duration of some walks if all is going well, and to add two elements. First, it's ideal, and perfectly safe, to boost your effort level during a couple of your walks each week, as long as you're feeling good and you're careful not to overheat or overexert. Just keep on eye on your heart rate, or Rate of Perceived Exertion—RPE (explained in chapter 1). Second, make some form of resistance training a routine part of your week.

GOALS FOR EACH WEEK

▪ Keep up your six-day-a-week (or more) walking average.

▪ Gradually add more minutes of walking, especially to your shorter-walk days. Build up so that 30 minutes is your daily minimum (other than when you don't feel good).

▪ By week 23, try to average one 60-minute walk (great for the weekend), two 40- to 50-minute walks, and three shorter walks per week.

▪ Pick up the pace. On days you feel good—but no more than twice a week—try easing the pace up just one tick for the middle 10 to 15 minutes of a walk. So if you normally walk at a 5 on the Rate of Perceived Exertion (RPE) 1-to-10 scale (chapter 1), boost to a 6 for the midsection of one or two walks.

▪ Still break up your walk time when necessary.

▪ Do the simple warm-ups before every walk and the full stretch routine after every walk you can. Use the quick stretch routine if time or space is limited. (All shown in chapter 3.)

▪ As soon as you feel up to it, add the simple strength routine two days a week. Over the course of the trimester, gradually try to build up to three days.

A TYPICAL WEEK IN MID-LATE TRIMESTER II, MODERATE PROGRAM:							
	MON.	**TUES.**	**WED.**	**THUR.**	**FRI.**	**SAT.**	**SUN.**
WALK (minutes)	45	30	35, 15 (PICK UP)	35	25	60 (PICK UP)	OFF
OTHER STUFF	WARM-UPS, FULL FLEX	WARM-UPS, QUICK STRETCH, STRENGTH	WARM-UPS, FULL FLEX	WARM-UPS	WARM-UPS, FULL FLEX, STRENGTH	WARM-UPS, QUICK STRETCH	

CHALLENGING PROGRAM, TRIMESTER II

You may be finding yourself champing at the bit to get back to your pre-pregnancy exercise routine. That's not unreasonable, as long as you keep in mind the changes your body is going through and the precautions we've outlined. Now is a good time to gradually increase the duration of your walks, and to boost the speed now and then. If you've done strength training before pregnancy, it's fine to continue that routine, or to do the strength routine we've outlined. In either case, take care to watch for warning signs that you're working too hard.

GOALS FOR EACH WEEK

- Keep walking six days a week or more.

- Add walking minutes. Over several weeks, boost your longest weekly walk (often easiest done on the weekend) to 75 minutes if you feel up to it, and gradually increase the length of two or three other weekly walks.

- By week 22, try to average one long walk (more than an hour), three 45- to 60-minute walks, and two 30- to 40-minute walks per week.

- Pick up the pace. On days you feel good—but no more than three times a week—try increasing the pace for the middle 15 to 30 minutes of a walk. So if you normally walk at a 5 on the Rate of Perceived Exertion (RPE) 1-to-10 scale (chapter 1), boost to a 6 or 7 for the midsection of two or three walks.

- Do the simple warm-ups before, and full stretch routine after, as many walks as possible (both are shown in chapter 3).

- If you did resistance exercise (such as lifting weights) before pregnancy, keep it up but at a lower intensity and with caution. It's important to eliminate or modify any exercises done lying on your back. If not, now is the time to add the simple strength routine described in this chapter. Begin doing it two days a week; after a few weeks, add a third day a week.

A TYPICAL WEEK IN MID-LATE TRIMESTER II, MODERATE PROGRAM:							
	MON.	TUES.	WED.	THUR.	FRI.	SAT.	SUN.
WALK (minutes)	60 (PICK UP)	30	45 (PICK UP)	35, 25	40 (PICK UP)	75	OFF
OTHER STUFF	WARM-UPS, FULL FLEX, STRENGTH	WARM-UPS, FULL FLEX	WARM-UPS, QUICK STRETCH, STRENGTH	WARM-UPS, FULL FLEX	WARM-UPS, FULL FLEX, STRENGTH	WARM-UPS, FULL FLEX	

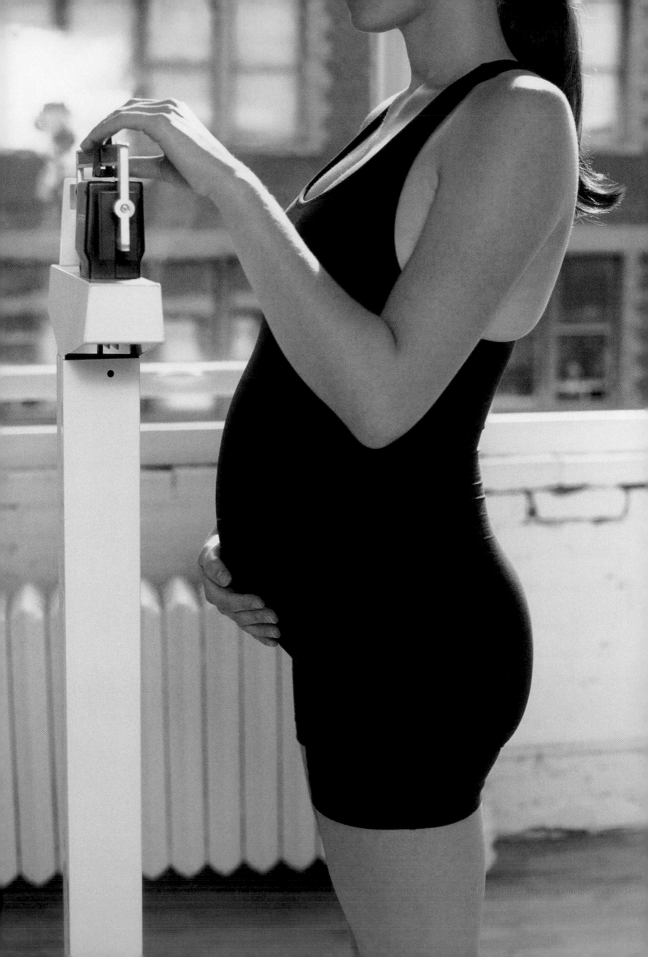

Don't Let Getting Big Get You Down

Walking to Delivery

You're in the home stretch now. With D-day drawing nearer, baby's ever-increasing size starts to have a much bigger effect on how you get around. With major developmental work done, her growth is more rapid now. By the end of this trimester, she'll stretch out to about 20 inches and weigh roughly six to nine pounds. The extra weight and size of your belly will affect you in several ways.

HERE COMES THE SLOW-DOWN

Expect it to slow you down naturally. "Even professional and Olympic athletes slow down at this point," says Dr. Raul Artal. "Put 20 pounds on the front of a healthy man, and he'd slow down, too." So don't fret if your steps are slower—it's perfectly normal. So is more soreness in the legs and hips, lower back, and shoulders with all the added weight. Though you may not be inclined to, it's important to maintain some strength routine and especially the stretches throughout this trimester to hold your posture together.

YOUR SHIFTING CENTER

As your belly grows, your center of mass shifts, making balance a more tricky proposition. That, combined with the fact that your joints are looser now (thanks to pregnancy hormones that loosen ligaments in anticipation of delivery), makes this a smart time to take care in choosing where you walk. You're more apt to fall, and more prone to injury if you do. So favor smooth paths and sidewalks, and be extra cautious when weather makes footing slick with rain, mud, ice, or snow.

This is a great time to switch to more supportive shoes; consider midcuts or high-tops, especially if you're feeling you can turn your ankles easily. (That's perfectly likely, with increasingly lax ligaments.) You really have two choices. Mid- or high-cut cross-training shoes still have an athletic feel, but offer a slightly wider base of support, and may be a bit stiffer than walking sneakers. That's a good trade for the increased stability.

An even better option is a rugged walking or light hiking shoe (different manufacturers use different terms). These have a slightly stiffer sole with a deeper tread, have a wider base, and are usually more "outdoorsy" looking than sneakers, with more color than white in the uppers. The best picks have a rounded or beveled heel to accommodate the rolling walking stride, and they're as comfy as any sneaker, but with greater support and stability. Opt for models without extra-thick treads on the outsole—you don't need a tripping hazard.

BABY TAKES UP MORE REAL ESTATE

Many women—even if they're fit—start to notice shortness of breath. As baby takes up more room, the uterus pushes up against the diaphragm, affecting your breathing. This might ease up late in the trimester, when baby drops down in preparation for delivery.

But there's a trade-off. As baby fills more space and drops lower, there will be more pressure on the bladder, sending you to the bathroom much more frequently.

CONTRACTIONS ON THE RISE

You may begin to have contractions. These may be the real deal, signaling the beginning of labor, or false alarms that range from a tightening across the abdomen to a more painful sensation. False, or Braxton-Hicks, contractions can be

kicked off by activity, and are more common when you're tired and closer to your due date. False contractions should stop if you do something different—sit instead of walk; walk instead of lying down—or change position. Real contractions come at regular intervals and get both stronger and closer together, no matter how you change your position or degree of activity.

EXERCISE IS STILL SAFE

You may be more aware of the baby's movement than ever—he's larger, and may be giving you real kicks in the ribs and elsewhere—but don't fret if he doesn't seem to move as much when you're exercising. Dr. Marjorie Meyer of UVM says that routine assessment of fetal movement (kick counts) has not been shown to be helpful or indicative of much. "When women are busy they feel less movement, and it's likely that exercise will distract the woman in the same manner. A better approach is to make sure you are well hydrated before and during exercise, and don't push yourself to the maximum capacity," she recommends. "Listen to how your body feels and stop when you feel dizzy or just plain bad." Of course, if you're concerned about decreased fetal movement, you should call your physician.

Finally, there's no truth to the old myth that exercise speeds up delivery, unless you're predisposed to premature delivery. Provided your pregnancy is not high risk or complicated, there's no reason you can't be one of those women who exercises right up until the day she delivers. Just know that to stay active and carry the fitness benefits you've worked hard for thus far, you'll need to make some adjustments. Exercise should leave you refreshed, not wiped out.

How Big Is Baby, Trimester III?

By 40 weeks, baby is approximately 20 inches long, and may weigh six to nine pounds.

Key developments: With lots of intricate developmental work done, it's time for some serious growing. Most babies gain three and a half to six and a half pounds during this trimester. Active babies deliver solid kicks, but tend to move less as their quarters get tight toward your due date. Late in the trimester, baby may drop into a lower, head-down position to get ready to exit.

What this means for you: Expect the extra weight to increase fatigue. Shortness of breath and more trips to the bathroom are common, as baby pushes on your diaphragm and bladder. Nighttime kicks may keep you up, exacerbating fatigue (but of course baby will sleep quietly when you walk or otherwise move around). And with delivery nearing, anticipate contractions, false or real.

Walking with Double the Weight

Sue Ryder, Sudbury, Massachusetts

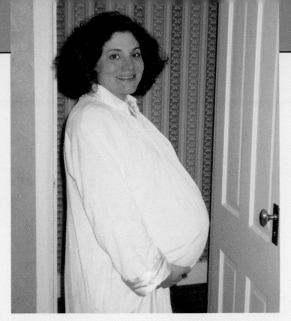

It took walking through pregnancy with twins to really light Sue Ryder's competitive fires. A mother of four boys—Jake (11), David (9), and twins Andrew and Nathan (5)—and freelance designer, Sue, above, spent more than 20 years in the athletic footwear industry. She knows the value of fitness, and worked out pretty regularly through her first two pregnancies, gaining only about 25 pounds each time. Her third pregnancy with the twins was a whole different story.

Within the first couple of months, she felt huge. Walking was her choice because she didn't have to commit a whole hour to a class. "Plus it was still warm, and I could use the time to enjoy the weather and contemplate the chaos my life was going to become with four kids," she fondly recalls. By six months, she was as big as she'd been at full term with the other two pregnancies. "I ended up with a 40-pound gain only because the twins were a few weeks early. I was heading to 50 for sure."

To keep moving late in pregnancy, Sue walked around a raised track at her community center. On Tuesday and Thursday, about 15 men and women from the retirement home would get dropped off by bus to use the center, and she recalls two women who were regulars. "I remember them perfectly because they were so striking. One had a neat gray ponytail tied with a black bow and the other had very short salt-and-pepper hair that was always perfect. They wore new white walking shoes and I thought, *Thank God I didn't design those,* because I always imagined my shoes being worn by beautiful college girls with coordinating outfits."

The ladies—both at least 80—didn't walk together, because one was clearly faster than the other. But Sue was hopeful when she saw them get off the bus the first day: "I thought I'd at least have the pleasure of passing *somebody* on the track. But salt-and-pepper lady must have thought that about me as well, as she not only passed me but lapped me and passed me again. The lady with the bow was more my pace but every time I got close to passing her, she'd pour on the juice. Some people are just so competitive." Why such athletic toughness? Sue says, "You could tell they didn't want to be passed by some giant huffing puffing pregnant lady."

Which leads her to ask, "Maybe I should send them some new sportier shoes?"

Thankfully, walking worked out well for Sue even as the weight piled on. "I walked up until I couldn't. My hips really hurt around the end. I was carrying so much weight and all my ligaments were so soft." But she always felt the walking helped and was glad to have a safe place to do it—even if the competition didn't cut her any slack.

WALKING IN THE THIRD TRIMESTER: HOW TO HANDLE THE INEVITABLE

THIRD-TRIMESTER SYMPTOMS	CAUSE	SOLUTION
Tendency to slow down	Baby is growing most rapidly now; you're carrying the greatest weight of pregnancy.	Move at your most natural pace; don't worry about slowing.
Shortness of breath	Uterus pushing on diaphragm.	Slow your pace, avoid hills; take multiple shorter walks instead of one longer.
Wobbly balance	Shifting center of mass.	Slow down, choose footing carefully, try high-top shoes.
Lax joints	Hormones are loosening ligaments that support joints.	Maintain low-resistance strength-training program (from chapter 6) as long as is comfortable.
Frequent need to urinate	Pressure on bladder from uterus and baby's weight.	Walk on a treadmill, mall, track—anywhere there's a bathroom nearby.
False contractions	Fatigue, physical activity.	Monitor contractions. Slow down or stop and rest.
Real contractions	Onset of labor.	If you're out walking, get home and time contractions to see if it's true labor.*

The American College of Obstetricians and Gynecologists say true labor is signaled by regular contractions that last from 30 to 70 seconds and start to occur more frequently.

Varicose Veins—A Reason to Keep Walking

First a warning—varicose veins are both hereditary and likely to get worse in each succeeding pregnancy. So if you know you're at risk, take notice and take all the precautionary measures you can. But what are they?

Arteries take oxygen-rich blood from your heart to your working muscles; veins bring the blue, oxygen-depleted blood back to the heart. There are one-way valves in the veins that help the blood return by keeping it from flowing backward in the veins. (See the one-way action by stroking a finger *away* from your heart along a visible vein in your forearm, and holding it near your wrist; release the finger, and watch the vein refill.)

Take It from Us:

Walking right up to the last minute

"After thinking I was mentally and physically prepped for the perfect, natural childbirth of Max, and then getting thrown a curve—a last minute c-section—I went into my second labor experience a little wiser. Dr. Evantash, my baby-faced obstetrician, had no qualms with me trying for a vaginal birth after cesarean (VBAC). My incision had healed normally, it had been over two years since my c-section, and I'd stayed fit by walking and lifting weights. He simply recommended the usual, "Stay hydrated and keep walking as long as you're comfortable—it helps urge the baby's head to naturally efface the cervix—and call me when it's time."

"Well, 'time' came two weeks early and predictably, since it was number two, we were nowhere near ready: no room, no bed, no name. At 7:00 A.M. while getting dressed for work my water broke. I'd walked the day before, and planned to walk that day—until that moment.

"We headed into the hospital where Dr. Evantash met us looking sixteen in his blue scrubs and shower cap (he noted it was a busy day for babies). I was examined—four centimeters dilated—and given there were no rooms available he said we should go for a little walk to keep things moving, music to Mark's ears. We strolled to lunch. By then I was just barely sensing contractions and was pretty cocky about the two block jaunt to the corner café. I hydrated with soup and lemonade and within about forty-five minutes could barely sit through a contraction without appearing obviously 'preoccupied.'The two blocks back seemed a lot longer, but at least by then I was quite sure the baby's head wasn't going to need a lot more "urging".

"We checked in, and found I was 10 centimeters dilated. Dr. Evantash hovered, Mark coached, and

I pushed. Mark knew from our training together not to be too chatty when I'm under duress so he held his tongue (for him, a feat akin to childbirth) while I focused. I knew there would be a little breather between pushes so I closed my eyes and tried to think of it

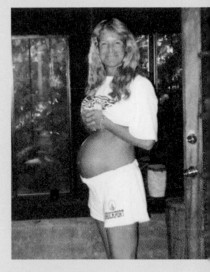

as breaks between my squat routines—only this was a competition and each push had to be my hardest. At one point between breaths, with Max's c-section very clear in my head, I asked Dr. Evantash if the baby was really coming out this way. He assured me I was only one 'strong' push away. Perhaps he was implying I was holding back, which, truth be told—well, I really had to dig deep given that it felt like I was about to blow out the whole bottom half of my body.

"Where the fitness and exercise paid off was getting through the tough part. I visualized being at the gym, with no spotter, maybe showing off a tad with one too many plates on my squat bar, and having absolutely no recourse but to push with all my might to get back up—or collapse in a pool of humiliation on the gym floor. The result: Skye was born, eight pounds, two ounces.

"Thankfully it was more hesitancy (okay, fear) than exhaustion that prolonged my labor. Lifting weights, pushing Max all around town in the jogger, and keeping up with the family walks right up until the end gave me the strength and endurance to come through it (relatively) unscathed.

—Lisa

✳TIP:

Keep hands,
feet, and
head warm
when cold
sets in. On
blustery days,
walk into the
wind first.

Several factors related to pregnancy can cause the valves to malfunction: the effect of tissue-relaxing hormones preparing your body for delivery, the increased pressure on the veins passing through the pelvis and abdomen, your expanded blood volume (supplying both you and baby), and simply the increase in weight and thus pressure on the legs. The result is a pooling of blood in the leg veins—in some cases they simply become more blue and spidery, but in others the veins can literally bulge on the leg's surface. Similarly, they can be quite painful and somewhat achy, or you might not feel them at all. The risk and severity of varicose veins can be reduced with the following measures.

THINGS TO AVOID:

▪ Excessive weight gain.

▪ Long periods of standing, sitting with your legs hanging, sitting cross-legged, or kneeling back on your heels.

▪ Straining during bowel movements.

▪ Restrictive clothing (other than support hose). For example, tight waistbands can further restrict blood return to the heart.

▪ Smoking—it has very bad effects on circulation.

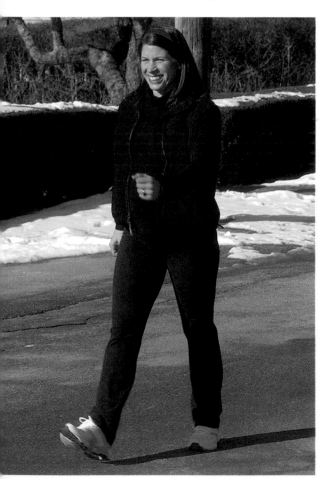

THINGS TO DO:

▪ Exercise! Walking is the best choice, creating gentle but consistent pumping action in the leg muscles. But gentle stretching and strength training help boost circulation, too.

▪ Maintain good nutrition—especially vitamin C to help keep veins healthy and elastic.

▪ Wear support panty hose. Frumpy or not, they can be a great help; put them on before getting out of bed and take them off at night before lying down.

For many women, the condition will clear up, or at least get better, as they return to their pre-pregnancy weight. And take comfort in knowing that regular walking will help both in prevention and in recovery.

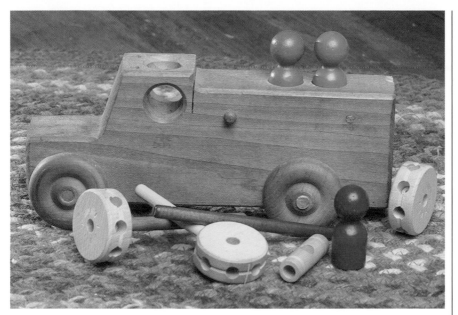

※**TIP:**

Know the
true value
of time,
snatch,
seize, and
enjoy every
moment
of it.

What to Do While Waiting for Baby

We asked lots of people for their best ideas regarding what to do as anxiety builds and you wait for labor to start. But rather than share all the predictable suggestions—paint the baby's room, write shower thank-you notes—we want to offer some thoughts from our colleague and friend Kevin Weafer. The former publisher of *Walking* magazine is a father of three, and though manly in all ways (hey, he works for *Men's Journal* and *Rolling Stone* now), he's most important a walker at heart, and a guy not afraid to get in touch with his feminine side. Thus, his ideas:

- Anything bird-related—watching, building houses for them, listening.
- Odd forms of dancing.
- Wondering "out loud."
- Ridiculous laughter.
- Read at least three to five of the greatest books ever written.
- Write poems to baby.
- Sporting events—"be" with others, ideally in the rafter seats.
- Buy clothing "while in a dream(y) state."
- Listening more carefully than ever.
- Practice being on the floor.
- Don't overthink the color thing.
- Own wooden stuff.

- Be away from electronic everything.
- Have your eyes closed as much as possible.
- Use colors loudly.
- Fidget freely.
- Make your way to snow.
- Pick up stones.
- Save the littlest things.
- Be fearless.
- Test-drive something.
- Buy a small appliance.
- Get a deeper peek at what makes you tick. Think.
- Ponder infinity.
- Use a telescope.
- Eat so much of something that you begin to laugh.

- Dawdle.
- Swing your arms fully.
- Rub your feet.
- Stock up on toys.
- Banish something from your life.
- Learn kid language.
- Smell hard.
- Twiddle your thumbs.
- Find a sentence that moves you.
- Try to move a marble on a table with your mind.
- Use the dictionary.
- Walk almost everywhere.

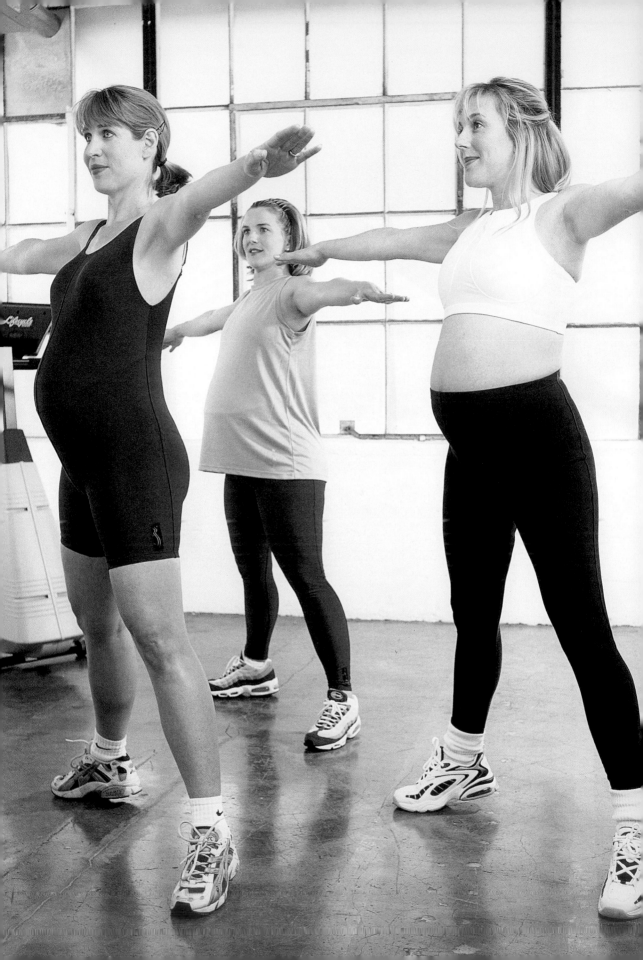

Gear 303: Getting Suited Up

8

Workout Wear for Pregnancy

When Lisa and Tracy were first pregnant, the pickings were slim when it came to maternity fitness clothing. You might have found cotton shorts or pants with a special wide band to support your belly, but you'd have to improvise the rest. Just six to eight years later, though, there's been an explosion of active wear for pregnant women. Both found working out a treat in their second pregnancies, with great pants that really fit and didn't fall off when they walked, and the same wicking tops that they couldn't live without before pregnancy, but now cut to fit a pregnant belly. These clothes weren't just supersized (and thus big all over); they really fit, they really moved with the body, and they were truly comfortable.

It's about time. Your husband's T-shirts don't cut it for workouts when you're not pregnant, so why should you have to wear them when you are? Here are five reasons it's worth investing in a few pieces of maternity workout apparel, even though it will have a short shelf life:

1. **FIT.** Try the old buy-a-size-bigger approach and you'll end up with gaping armholes and clothing that binds in some places but droops in others. Well-designed maternity workout clothing is specifically cut to fit and expand with a woman's pregnant shape.

2. **SUPPORT.** Many of the tops and bottoms you'll find have padding or extra panels to add support—a big deal when your belly and breasts get heavy and your back is taking a beating.

3. **MOISTURE MANAGEMENT.** Clammy, damp cotton tees are history. Today's maternity fitness clothing is made from technical fabrics that draw sweat and moisture away from your skin to help it evaporate. You stay drier, cooler, and more comfortable.

4. **LOOKS.** Some styles are decidedly hip, others more conservative. Either way, there's a look that suits you and won't make you feel like you're relegated to someone else's old gray sweats just because you're having a baby.

5. **COMFORT.** More and more manufacturers are paying attention to details, like smooth seams that won't irritate a tender belly. And because every body's different, there are even options such as bottoms that sit above or below the belly. Comfort happens when you get the right fit, support, details, fabric, and looks, and with comfort, you may be more likely to stick with exercise through your pregnancy. By the same token, uncomfortable gear will only irritate you and give you one more reason to opt for a big comfy chair.

GOOD QUESTION

How do I pick clothes for being active (while steering clear of the tent Omar made me)?

We surveyed current and past active pregnant women regarding their favorite pregnancy duds. The "older crowd" (authors included) had decidedly low-tech answers, while the younger set had more experience with the newer apparel offerings. Some of their thoughts:

- "Leotards and sweats—especially zip-front sweat-shirts."
- "Maternity belt for my back."
- "Exercise tights, a well-supporting bra, and an oversized buttondown shirt from Roger's closet."
- "Stretch pants in basic colors. I stayed away from trendy and overpriced maternity apparel. Went for casuals and basics in comfort materials like T-shirt cottons and fleece, then I could dress them up or down depending on my schedule."
- "Winter pregnancy, so mittens/gloves were vital. Also the shoe and pant thing needed to be right."
- "Stretch pants with stirrups and comfortable sneakers."
- "For swimming: bathing suit (regular bikini works fine), goggles."
- "Bike shorts with a low, giant, wide waistband that I could position under Junior so it didn't feel like he was going to drop right out of my stomach."

- "White, supercushioned midcut aerobic shoes with fluffy padded socks. Loose, knit athletic shorts that I could roll down under my belly and a giant T-shirt to cover it all."

Bottom Line: Comfort is king! The most sophisticated of the crowd focused on functional sweat management (wicking, quick-dry blends) and ease around an expanding belly for workout gear, while many enjoyed comfort fabrics (cotton, fleece) for general wear.

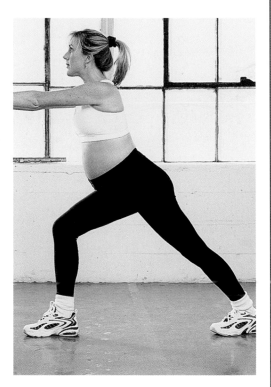

THE OPTIONS: You name it, it's out there. Sports bras (and active nursing bras), tank tops, tops with various sleeve lengths, shorts and pants of every length and cut, unitards, leotards, swimsuits, and more are all available.

UPSIDE: Comfort, comfort, comfort means you'll enjoy and look forward to workouts.

DOWNSIDE: Shelling out cash for gear that you use for a limited time. (But do hang on to it for the next pregnancy, or your sister's . . .)

LOOK FOR: Basic pieces in solid colors. If you don't mind frequent laundry, you can probably work with a minimum of one or two supportive bras, a pair of shorts or pants (depending on the climate and season), and two tops.

BRANDS INCLUDE: Belly Basics, Fit Maternity, Liz Lange for Nike, Mothers in Motion, The Power of Two by adidas, Reebok.

Layering It On in Any Season

As you get heavier and delivery closes in, you've got to minimize any possible barriers to getting out the door and walking. Feeling too hot or cold, especially in your hypersensitive state, will be a surefire turnoff to taking a walk. So build a walking wardrobe—just a few key pieces—to help keep your walking on track.

THE BOTTOM LAYER—
CLOSEST TO YOUR SKIN

Whether it's hot or cold, the best starters are undergarments of wicking materials such as CoolMax or polypropylene. They transport moisture away from your skin, keeping you from feeling drenched on hot and humid days, and avoiding a damp chill in winter. More and more sports bras are available in the same moisture-wicking fabrics—some are supportive and discreet enough that it's all some women wear in very hot weather. When it comes to undies, avoid anything with itchy tags and tight spots.

THE MIDDLE LAYER—SHIRTS AND PANTS

Cotton sweatpants and shirts are a thing of the past for real exercise. Suitable only for a dry cool day and a low-intensity walk, if they get wet (from sweat or rain) they get heavy, uncomfortable, and—worse—they provide no insulation. Think of microfibers and other quick-dry blends for shorts and shirts in warmer weather, and synthetic fleece tops and bottoms in cooler conditions. Fleeces come in a variety of weights (from light jerseys and sweaters to heavy zip-front jackets and pullovers) and styles ranging from sleek body-conforming stretch pants to downright baggy sweats.

THE OUTER LAYER—WIND AND RAIN

The need for outer layers means it's either cold, wet, windy, or all three. For cold, synthetic fleece materials (often called Polarfleece) are the best insulating materials going. They're light, comfortable, and warm even if wet. You can soak a fleece jacket in water, then squeeze and shake it out and

wear it, and feel insulated. It will be damp, but it's vastly better than a soaked cotton sweatshirt, which is essentially useless. If you don't have any fleece, then the original insulating-when-wet alternative—wool—is a choice, as long as you don't have a problem with itching.

When wind and rain are threats, high-tech fabrics such as Gore-Tex and its many cousins are ideal. They shed rain but allow sweat in the form of water vapor to escape the fabric, and are designed in everything from light wind jackets to full parkas with down insulation. But don't fret if you don't own such fancy outerwear. For a 30-minute walk, a decent nylon windbreaker over your insulating layer will usually suffice in breaking the wind and withstanding drizzle. In heavier rain, consider a good old rubberized slicker; you can get a rain jacket and pants for

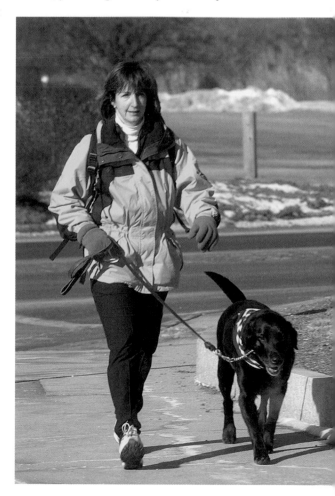

less than $50, and they keep you from using rain as an excuse not to take a walk. But it's not breathable, and on a longer or faster walk your own sweat may dampen you from the inside.

SOCKS

After shoes, decent socks are the next most important investment you can make. Go with synthetic blends, or some of the high-quality wool socks woven with a super-soft feel (see "Socks" in the resource list); try models with slightly thicker padding in the heel and ball of the foot. Cotton socks seem comfortable when warm and dry, but as you sweat they bunch up, lose cushioning, and can even cause blisters.

Walking with Poles—The Next Trend?

Carrying hand weights went through a brief surge of popularity among walkers looking to boost their workouts, though lately the fad appears to have waned. But the real hot trend in exercise walking in the United States may be just around the corner. Walking with poles is a new rage in Finland and it's spreading into other European countries. Of course, the Finns have an amazing tradition of cross-country or Nordic skiing, and in deference they've christened their new summertime fitness fad *Nordic walking*.

Though we don't have such deep Nordic roots in the United States, and perhaps a higher sensitivity to looking goofy in public, we've also been quick to embrace new exercise ideas, even contrived ones, if they work. (Think Step and Spinning classes—need we say more?) And the idea of walking with poles is surprisingly on-target for pregnant women, because they can add stability when you're least sure-

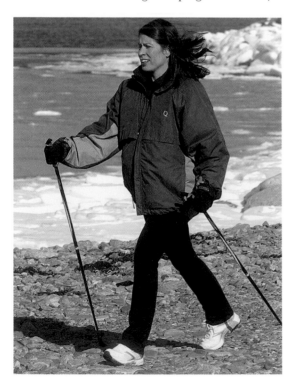

footed, they provide a bit of an upper-body workout to a walk, and they may reduce some of the loads on overworked hip, knee, and ankle joints.

HOW IT'S DONE: The arm movement is really the same as the poling motion during the classical (traditional, or diagonal) cross-country skiing stride. Your right arm swings forward and plants the pole just as your left foot hits the ground, and vice versa.

THE OPTIONS: You can go with the old cross-country ski poles in the closet, but that leaves you with metal tips that grate and slip on asphalt, and unneeded baskets near the pole tips (designed to keep the pole on top of the snow) that just get in the way. Instead, consider one of the two types of poles specifically designed for walkers.

Trekking poles are usually adjustable-length (telescoping, with twist locks) aluminum poles, so you can shorten them for carrying on your pack when hiking on level ground. They're designed for maintaining balance on rough ground and easing the burden of carrying a heavy pack on trails.

Exercise or Nordic walking poles are fixed length, generally made of lighter and more durable composite materials, and have removable rubber tips and fancier handgrips. They're intended for use anywhere—from trails to sidewalks—by anyone hoping to boost the intensity and upper-body benefits of a walking workout.

UPSIDE: Plenty of benefits to your workout, including:

- Improved balance and security.
- Enhanced upper-body workout. Low resistance work for back, chest, shoulders, triceps (back of the upper arms).
- Easily adjustable intensity—pole vigorously, or just place them for support.
- Reduced joint strain. Lessens impact on feet and force transmitted to knees, ankles, and hips by putting some load onto the poles, arms, and shoulders.

DOWNSIDE: You have to store the poles, and you may feel silly at first. But head out onto a paved trail where everyone else is doing their own thing, too (in-line skating, racewalking, riding tandem and recumbent bikes), and you'll just feel like part of the latest exercise trend.

LOOK FOR: Comfortable handgrips. Adjustable wrist straps are a must, so you can release the pole at the end of each pushing stroke. Removable rubber tips—use them on pavement, remove them on grass or dirt trails.

BRANDS INCLUDE: Exel, Exerstrider for fitness walking; Leki for trekking poles.

TIP:
Walking uphill increases the intensity of your walk, even if you slow down a bit; the steeper the hill, the greater the intensity.

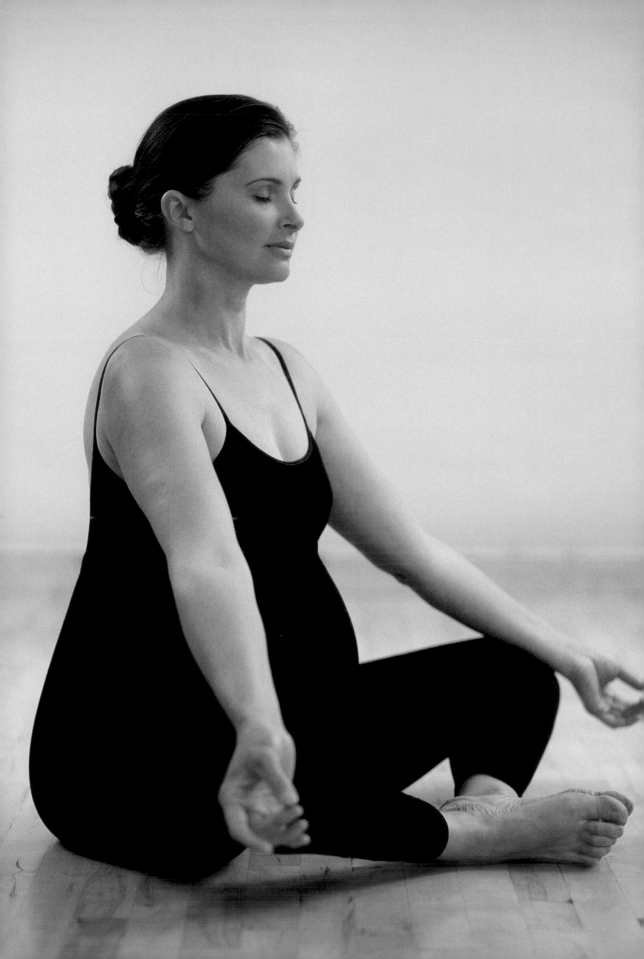

Walking to Delivery Time

Trimester III

Now it's time for the payoff. You've (hopefully) had six months of building reliable activity habits following our recommendations. If you've exercised religiously and your experience lines up with the research, your weight gain has been at a healthy pace, you haven't struggled horribly with fatigue and discomfort, and you're feeling fairly strong, fit, and even resilient. Though you may not realize it, the greatest reward is coming now—the fact that even as you get larger, you'll have the strength, flexibility, and endurance to get through these final weeks and the delivery with flying colors.

Yoga for Relaxation in the Home Stretch

It seems yoga is the latest trend among the health club set. But advocates will point out that yoga is anything but a recent fad; it's just that many Americans are only now discovering the beauty and balance of this holistic exercise. And it's fast becoming a favorite among pregnant women. Why? One thing that sets yoga apart from other exercises is the strong connection to breathing, according to Colette Crawford, RN, master yoga instructor and founder of the Seattle Holistic Center.

"One type of breathing is Ujjayi breathing, or victorious breathing. The sound of the breath helps the mind to focus on one point, which helps the woman to be in the present moment," says Crawford. "It also balances energy; it can help her to access her energy as well. We know that energy cannot be created or destroyed, but it can get stuck. Ujjayi and doing yoga postures helps to free this energy."

That may seem a little abstract or crunchy if you've never done yoga before, but any woman who's attended even the most traditional birthing class knows controlled breathing during labor is strongly recommended. Birthing partners are even coached to count during slow, deep breaths. So practicing before delivery seems pretty logical.

But it's not just about breathing—many yoga postures can help alleviate common discomforts of pregnancy. "Yoga can help with sciatica, restless legs, low back pain, pelvic pain, neck and should pain, even heartburn and nausea," points out Crawford. "Yoga poses can also help a woman strengthen and build endurance without strain." And she asserts the whole-person approach of yoga better prepares a woman for the challenge of delivery. "Birth is a physical as well as emotional and spiritual experience. Yoga connects all those aspects of being human. Knowing your state of mind and learning not to attach yourself to it allows the body to do what it needs to do."

She suggests practicing the following Ujjayi breathing ("victorious breathing") during stretching or ideally yoga, and then being able to call on the skill during labor.

- Part your lips slightly, inhale and exhale whispering "ahh." You'll feel and hear the breath in the back of the throat. Then close your mouth and breathe through the nostrils. Imagine saying "sa" as you inhale and "ha" as you exhale. Your breath will have an aspirant sound. If you feel any strain, breathe normally before continuing.
- After the birth, use Ujjayi breathing often to relax, recover, and re-energize. Lie on your back with knees bent, or sit comfortably with your spine erect and head in line with your back. Repeat the breathing pattern just described, first with open mouth, then through your nostrils. Keep your attention on the breathing, bringing it back when your mind wanders. This helps create focus and calm, and can be done anytime, including while nursing.

GOOD QUESTION

Is my fitness going to help me get through labor and delivery?

You've probably been reading books or attending classes in anticipation of labor and delivery, and so have a sense of what you're in for. If not, we recommend you do, because we know of many women (including two of the authors) who felt that knowing what was coming, and bringing an athlete's mind-set to the process, aided delivery tremendously. There are three stages. The first is where your body (and pain threshold) pretty much do all the work without you; you just have to ride it out. This stage is, in turn, separated into three phases:

1. Early phase. Contractions are mild to moderate, and it can take from a few hours to two weeks; some women don't even know it's happening. But if you do, this is where endurance training will pay off. Walking six days a week and taking occasional longer walks have built your overall conditioning and stamina to work through this bearable, but sometimes very long, buildup.

2. Active phase. Shorter than the first, contractions are stronger, longer, and more frequent; you should be at the hospital now. The faster, more intense walks and your strength training pay off here. Though this phase is challenging, it's shorter, and

you may be able to look at each hard contraction as just another hard part of your workout.

3. Transitional. The most demanding and exhausting part of labor. Intensity spikes, and contractions are fast and furious; you often can't tell when one is over and the next starts. But it only averages 15 minutes to an hour long, so this is where your hardest workouts may help. If you've got toughness in reserve, this is when you'll call it up. It may be harder than anything you've done before, but you're fit and strong and will survive.

In the second stage of labor, called (surprise) delivery, you get pushing and the baby arrives. This will require explosive bursts of strength as you push, and quick recovery between contractions. But at least you're done waiting, and all your strength and stretching work may actually help. So will having a good sense of your body and believing in your own fitness. And though you may be exhausted, rest assured that you'll be less exhausted than if you hadn't put in all the work you put in while pregnant. (The third and final stage is called delivery of the placenta—anticlimactic, but an important wrap-up to your effort.)

Bottom Line: Nothing will guarantee a smooth or pain-free labor and delivery, but most women who've exercised through pregnancy attest to the benefit of being fit and strong for this, one of life's greatest and most rewarding events.

"Feet, Don't Fail Me Now"

Cathy Robinson, Boston, Massachusetts

Cathy, a graphic artist and mother of Yasmine (3), and Jared (1), has always been a believer in walking, though she admits having little choice. She grew up with athletic parents (Dad still insists on a tennis game when they get together), she played competitive tennis through college, and she spent years as assistant art director at *Walking*, a national health and fitness magazine. With that pedigree, you can imagine her concern when she started experiencing lots of swelling and mild varicose veins during her first pregnancy.

"My feet and ankles got really swollen," she says. "I called them tree trunks. And my ankles looked really weird. I actually lost sight of the bones; they were just gone." But it wasn't just the appearance of swelling—the ankles actually felt physically stiff. "*Turgid* is the word that comes to mind." That left walking anything but comfortable. "Even after a short walk to lunch, they'd be aching," she recalls. "It was a throbbing feeling, and the skin was stretched so tight that it was sensitive to the touch."

Dealing with Swollen Feet

She struggled to get her feet into any shoes during the last trimester. "I had one pair of wide athletic shoes, and a pair of comfy Rockport zip-up midcut shoes that were all I wore. The midcut gave a bit more support," she says with a laugh, "and the zip front was nice because I didn't have to lean over to tie them."

During her second pregnancy, Cathy started right from the beginning all the preventive measures she could to reduce the swelling and varicose veins, including:

■ Minimizing the time sitting with her feet hanging down. She got ergonomic foot rests, to comfortably raise her feet when sitting at the desk.

■ Never crossing her legs when sitting.

■ Making a conscious effort to move often throughout the day; she'd go up and down the stairs, walk rather than send an e-mail, pace while on the phone.

■ Trying to drink a lot more water—she'd been told it would help to flush the system—and get up often to refill.

■ Putting her feet up when she got home (and asking husband Darryl for a gentle foot massage).

In the end, the key to staying active for Cathy—both during her pregnancies and now with children—has been working walking into the day. "It's not necessarily about exercise walks. I do errands on foot—even just 10 minutes at a time—because working downtown I could go to the pharmacy, post office, lunch on foot."

Will She Have Surgery for the Varicose Veins?

Cathy read about surgery and laser treatments, but felt it was too experimental. She still has mild varicose veins, but they're not painful and she feels it's not worth messing with them. "I can cover them with knee-length skirts. I was always more of a pants chick anyway.

"Plus," she adds, "I view my body very differently now. My focus is on the kids, not myself." She admits that as an athlete, her condition was very important to her. "You admired yourself. But now you know your hips won't be as skinny, you'll never have quite as flat a six-pack belly again. For me varicose veins is part of the package. Sure, I'll be different." But is that a problem for Cathy? On the contrary, she considers it a small price to pay.

The Third-Trimester Walking Program

GENERAL REMINDERS FOR TRIMESTER III

Don't give up the ship! This is the time when everything from varicose veins to swollen ankles may have you wondering what you've gotten yourself into. But now more than ever, daily walks are key to staying healthy and sane, and even sleeping better.

- Be flexible. As your body finishes off its internal project, you'll really have to adjust your daily workouts to how you feel—some days you'll plow through the recommended walk, some days nothing close.

- Now it's more important than ever: If anything feels wrong or discomfort persists, back off and check with your doctor.

- Become the master of the multiwalk day. As you get large enough to feel you have your own gravitational pull, you may find you simply don't want to be on your feet for an hour at a

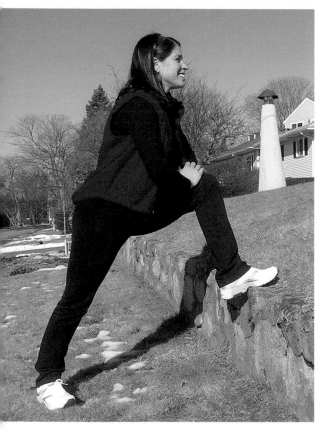

time. But you'll also discover that short walks really help relieve ankle swelling, lower-back tightness, and the *I-can't-get-comfortable-in*-any-*position* blues. Going for as many as four or five shorter walks over the day will help you feel better and maintain your hard-won fitness. Plus, shorter walks keep you close to home in case you have to cut things short.

- Use the warm-ups and stretch routine to maintain comfort. You'll probably find that even if you're not going for a walk, a few minutes of the warm-up routine followed by one or two strength and stretching moves (say, pelvic tilt, shoulder stretch) can get the blood flowing, ease stiffness or fatigue, and help you feel better. In other words, get up and move, get down and stretch.

- Warm up daily—we won't show it on the program anymore, but do it before every walk, and whenever else you need it.

- Keep at those Kegels. If you've been doing these religiously, you're sick of Kegel exercises by now. But trust the women who've come before you—you're going to be happy you've been doing these a week after delivery when you actually still have some bladder control.

AN IMPORTANT NOTE

We've been saying all along that you have to listen to your body, but now that's more true than ever. Here's why: Some women will follow this program exactly, doing all we recommend and more right up until the day they deliver. (Think of Wendy Sharp paddling her kayak on delivery day!) Others may literally be put under restrictions by their doctors—in rare cases, even on bedrest during the final phase of pregnancy. This isn't something to fear, it's just an acknowledgment of the wide range of possibilities facing you. So enjoy the walking you can do, don't fret over what you can't, and appreciate your remaining days of calm.

LOW-KEY PROGRAM, TRIMESTER III

The key now is to listen to your body (and your doctor). Continue to walk every day, but be prepared for your walks to become less like formal exercise outings and more like activity that you sprinkle throughout the day. When feeling good, you should still maintain the length and intensity of the walks you've been doing. But don't be frustrated by a gradual but inexorable decrease in the speed of your walks and the distance you can cover. You're carrying more and more weight, and frankly most of it's not in a particularly convenient location, from the standpoint of walking efficiency. Still, as long as it's comfortable, you can try to maintain the *time* that you spend walking, even if it's broken up over the day, and a lot slower than before. But accept that as your due date approaches, even this may be a challenge.

GOALS FOR A TYPICAL WEEK

▪ Stick with your average of six walking days per week.

▪ Hold at your current distance and intensity for as long as it's comfortable. But be prepared to gradually reduce the distance and speed of your walks, following how you feel as a guide.

▪ Plan to break up more and more of your walks over the course of the day. Lots of short walks are just as good as one longer one—and possibly better, because they provide some variety and relief throughout the day.

▪ Use the warm-up routine anytime you think it will help you loosen up or ease discomfort (say, if your back or shoulders are feeling tight).

▪ Do the full stretch routine (chapter 3) two or three days a week, being careful not to strain or cause any discomfort. Expect your range of motion to be reduced as your belly fills out. Use the quick stretch routine if it's easier or more comfortable to stay standing.

A TYPICAL WEEK IN MID-LATE TRIMESTER III, LOW-KEY PROGRAM:							
	MON.	TUES.	WED.	THUR.	FRI.	SAT.	SUN.
WALK (minutes)	10, 15	10	20	10, 10	15	10, 10, 10	OFF
OTHER STUFF	FULL FLEX		QUICK STRETCH	QUICK STRETCH		FULL FLEX	

MODERATE PROGRAM, TRIMESTER III

The challenge now is not to walk faster or farther, but to maintain your daily minutes of physical activity for as long as it's comfortable. Don't be fixated on your pre-pregnancy or even Trimester II abilities. Just listen to your body, do what you can when you can. Don't abandon the warm-ups, after-walk stretching, and light weight training as long as you can stick with them—all will help you feel much better than if you give up entirely. And maintaining your routine as long as possible now will help when it comes to post-partum fitness rebuilding.

GOALS FOR EACH WEEK

▪ Stick with your average of six walking days per week.

▪ Hold at your current distance and intensity for as long as it's comfortable. Be prepared to gradually reduce the distance and speed of your walks, but expect some days to be better than others.

▪ Pick up the pace or go longer when you feel good; back off when you don't.

▪ Break up more and more of your walks over the course of the day. Lots of short walks are just as good as one longer one—and possibly better, because they provide some physical variety and relief throughout the day.

▪ Use the warm-up routine anytime you think it will help you loosen up or ease discomfort (say, if your back or shoulders are feeling tight).

▪ Do the full stretch routine (chapter 3) two or three days a week, being careful not to strain or cause any discomfort. Expect your range of motion to be reduced as your belly fills out. Use the quick stretch routine if it's easier or more comfortable to stay standing.

A TYPICAL WEEK IN MID-LATE TRIMESTER III, MODERATE PROGRAM:							
	MON.	**TUES.**	**WED.**	**THUR.**	**FRI.**	**SAT.**	**SUN.**
WALK (minutes)	45	30	25, 15	35	25	50	OFF
OTHER STUFF	FULL FLEX	QUICK STRETCH, STRENGTH	FULL FLEX		FULL FLEX, STRENGTH	QUICK STRETCH	

CHALLENGING PROGRAM, TRIMESTER III

"Challenging" program or not, this is no time for heroics. Your biggest concern for this final trimester is maintaining an activity level that keeps you feeling healthy and comfortable, not one that proves you're a superjock. So forget about trying to increase your speed or distance. Instead, a healthy approach is to maintain your daily minutes of physical activity for as long as it's comfortable, and then begin a modest step-down that's in line with how you feel. One way to do this is to believe that it all will come back. If you've been sticking with the challenging program, you've maintained a great level of fitness.

GOALS FOR EACH WEEK

▪ Keep walking six days a week or more.

▪ Maintain your walking minutes for as long as is comfortable. Rather than mixing much longer (75 minutes) and shorter (30 minutes) walks, consider evening out your totals.

▪ Forget about speed. On days you feel good, you can pick up the pace a bit, but don't feel a need to ever push above an RPE of 6 this late in the game.

▪ Always do the simple warm-ups before, and full stretch routine after (both chapter 3), as many walks as possible.

▪ Stick with Kegel exercises whenever you think of it.

▪ Keep doing resistance (strength) exercises only as long as they're comfortable.

A TYPICAL WEEK IN MID-LATE TRIMESTER III, CHALLENGING PROGRAM:							
	MON.	**TUES.**	**WED.**	**THUR.**	**FRI.**	**SAT.**	**SUN.**
WALK (minutes)	25, 25	35	45	25, 20	30	60	OFF
OTHER STUFF	FULL FLEX, STRENGTH	FULL FLEX	QUICK STRETCH, STRENGTH	FULL FLEX	QUICK STRETCH, STRENGTH	FULL FLEX	

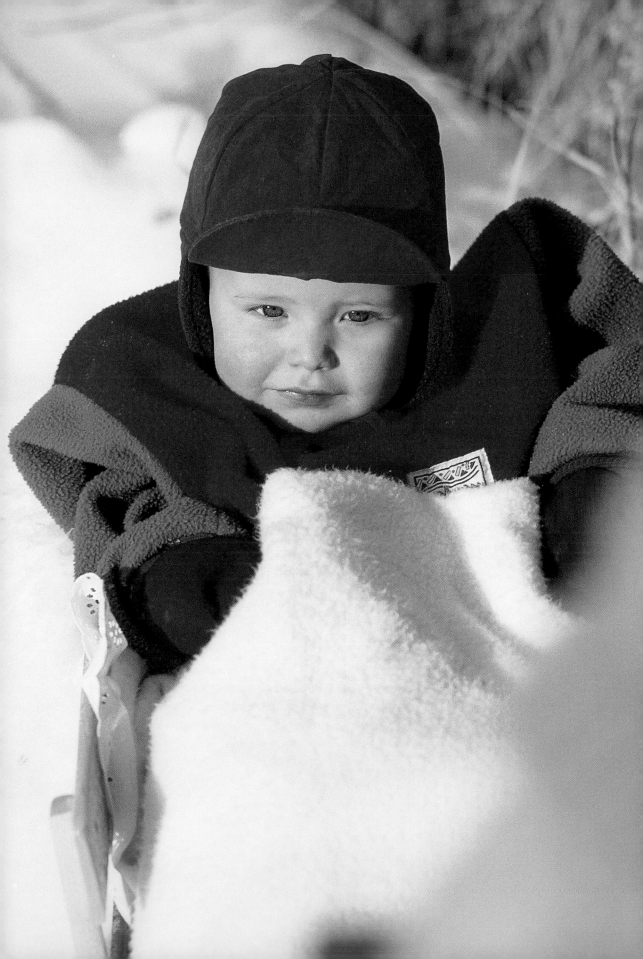

Exercise? Are You Kidding? I Haven't Brushed My Teeth in a Week.

Why Should You Keep Moving?

With a body that's just been through an amazing physical feat, a new baby to care for, and a sleep pattern that's as predictable as New England weather ("Don't like it? Just wait a minute . . ."), it's easy to see how exercise might be about as appealing to you right now as facing labor all over again. But it's more important than ever to keep your walking shoes busy. The deck may seem stacked against you, but exercise is actually your ally for feeling better in both the short and long term.

First, the big picture. Women who gain weight after delivery and women who exercise less after baby arrives than they did during pregnancy are both more likely to gain weight over the long term, reports Michelle Mottola, PhD, director of the R. Samuel McLaughlin Foundation Exercise and Pregnancy Laboratory at the University of Western Ontario. Add the fact that being overweight increases the risk for major health threats such as heart disease, diabetes, cancer, and a host of chronic afflictions and you can see why it's critical to continue the active patterns you've established already.

But weight loss isn't the only benefit. Physical inactivity is known to be a risk factor for chronic disease and early death, independent of whether you're overweight or not. In fact, in a series of major studies at the Cooper Institute in Dallas and at Harvard University, leading a sedentary lifestyle was found to increase your health risks about as much as smoking does. So not only can being active help get you to a healthy weight, but in and of itself a daily walk is good for you, even if you don't lose a pound. The 1996 *Surgeon General's Report on Physical Activity and Health* summed it up pretty concisely by recommending that every adult accumulate at least 30 minutes of moderate-intensity activity most (if not all) days of the week to assure a longer, healthier life. This at a time when, aside from smoking, the root causes of the greatest number of deaths in America are sedentary living and poor nutrition.

If the long-term health reasons don't move you to action, a more immediate concern might: fatigue. Around-the-clock feedings and the stress of trying to decipher which cry means what add up to one thing: You're more tired now than you've ever thought possible. And it won't end soon. In this state, overdoing it physically can make you more tired, but small doses of activity and short walks have the uplifting effect of a Starbucks Frappuccino. Getting active will energize you, lift your spirits, and help you get through a challenging time. Finally, exercise encourages healing in the abdominal, pelvic, and uterine muscles, and helps tighten up ligaments around joints that loosened up during pregnancy.

Exercise is also the smartest way to tackle an issue that's big on the mind of every new mom: getting your body back. Though all of the weight you put on during pregnancy hasn't magically melted off with the birth of your baby, this is no time for the South Beach Diet. Your body is working hard to recover, keep up with the demands of a baby's schedule, and, in many cases, produce milk around the clock. "If you're breast-feeding, you need a minimum of 1,800 kilocalories a day," says Mottola. "Try to ignore the scale, and instead get in tune with how you feel."

How Big Is Baby, Postmester I (0–3 months)?

Babies grow at different rates, but most weigh between 5 and 10 pounds at birth and may grow to 16 pounds by three months.

Key milestones: For the first several weeks, it's all about feeding and sleeping. Personality and developmental rates both vary widely, but many newborns settle into a more predictable pattern by about eight weeks. Your reward for what may be a tumultuous time: baby's first smile, between four and six weeks. Young infants focus best on objects that are about 12 inches away, and by three months most can focus on a toy or object that moves from side to side in front of them. As baby gains strength, she can lift her head off the mattress or floor when placed on her tummy, generally by two months. At this same time, baby starts to notice the outside world.

What this means for you: Nap when baby naps if you're tired, especially in the first few weeks. When you feel up to it, take advantage of naptime to take walks. Since young babies sleep so much of the time, that means you have lots of flexibility on when to go for a walk. A front carrier that supports baby's head and neck can be a godsend, freeing hands, soothing a fussy baby, and giving you another option for mobility in addition to the stroller (see chapter 11). When you notice baby taking an interest in his surroundings, he'll enjoy outings as a chance to take in the scenery, not just for the comforting motion.

A safer way to start regaining your prepregnancy shape is through exercise, which delivers the bonus of adding muscle and improving the efficiency of your heart and lungs. It also reduces your chances of continuing to gain weight, which is a real risk once the baby arrives. One Swedish study followed 1,423 women for a year after they delivered their babies and found that women who were inactive or more sedentary gained an average of 10 pounds or more by the end of that year, compared with women who were active. (Incidentally, put to rest any concerns that exercise might be a turnoff to nursing babies who dislike the sour taste caused by lactic acid. "The latest research shows that it's not an issue, unless you're doing exhaustive exercise," says Mottola.)

Now that you know why it's important to stick with exercise, how can you make it happen? Mottola's research shows that the two biggest keys for new moms are finding ways to exercise with baby and getting social support. Because child care is a biggie, it's all the better if you can adapt by taking baby along in a stroller or carrier, and learn new strengthening routines that let baby safely join in. Your partner can help in countless ways—by taking care of the baby, by getting up a little earlier or sharing chores to free up time for you to exercise, and by offering encouragement. "Lack of time and fatigue are also factors," adds Mottola. "But both social support and finding ways to exercise with baby can help you overcome these, too."

WHAT CAN YOUR BODY HANDLE NOW?

If you've had a normal, complication-free delivery, it's fine to start reintroducing activity as soon as you feel up to it. "I had a patient recently who wanted to stop at the gym on the way home from the hospital," said Raul Artal, MD, professor and chairman of the Department of Obstetrics, Gynecology, and Women's Health at the St. Louis University School of Medicine. "That's the most extreme I've seen, because really, labor can be

GOOD QUESTION

When can I really start exercising normally again?

About six weeks after baby arrives, you'll visit your doctor for a postpartum checkup, and that's the real time to answer this question. Though you've probably been able to take regular walks well before this point, this visit is the time to get clearance for stepping up your walking and a more formal exercise program. For the postpartum visit, do the following:

Be Prepared to Tell Your Doctor

- Whether or not you're breast-feeding.
- Whether you are still experiencing vaginal bleeding and how much.
- If you had a C-section, whether you're experiencing any soreness and in what situations.
- What activities you'd like to do for exercise.
- What foods you're eating and the amount of water you're drinking.

Be Sure to Ask Your Doctor

- Whether you need to take a nutritional supplement or continue taking prenatal vitamins. (If you're breast-feeding, you may need calcium and B_6 supplements to keep up with demands of exercise and lactation on top of limited sleep.)
- If there are any limitations on activities or duration of activity, provided that you increase the length and intensity of any physical activity gradually.
- What would be a safe rate of weight loss for you.

Bottom Line: By six weeks postpartum, most women can safely ramp up their exercise program, but it's important to discuss the details with your doctor first. Discuss postdelivery recovery, how you're feeling, your sleep and nutritional habits, any special concerns, and your fitness and weight loss goals. Then you can agree on a safe and healthy approach.

like running a marathon, and then, do you really want to run the day after that? Let your body be your guide." The guidelines below can help you get a safe start.

If you had a Cesarean section or a difficult delivery, expect it to take a bit more time before you feel strong enough, and your practitioner may have specific instructions for you about how much you can do, and when. If you had a normal delivery:

- Taking your baby for a walk is fine as soon as you're ready, and it's good to establish the habit for you and baby right away.

- Stretching, Kegels, and relaxation exercises are safe to do right away. Start abdominal exercises very slowly and progress gradually. Avoid any moves involving torque.

- Listen to your body, and use fatigue as your guide on how much activity to do. Don't overdo it. Taking brief rests as you walk can help you get going comfortably.

- Even if you exercised through your pregnancy, start back slowly, and gradually ramp up pace and distance.

The Big Benefits of Regular Exercise for New Moms

- Helps you get back to your pre-pregnancy shape.
- It's a safe, effective way to lose extra pregnancy weight, especially if you're breast-feeding.
- Increases energy at a time when you're more tired than ever.
- Boosts mood and helps you handle stress.
- Can reduce the likelihood that you'll struggle with postpartum depression.
- Reduces your risk for heart disease (the number one killer of women in America), breast cancer (a number one fear) and other cancers, diabetes, osteoporosis, hypertension, and early death.
- Provides a positive role model for your baby, which has been shown to help children be more active.

Take It from Us:

Two weeks since you gave birth, and you're still walking like you're on eggshells? Don't worry, you're no wimp!

I was tall and fit and was told by everyone from my doctor to my milkman how easy my labor would be. 'Oh, one push and he'll shoot right out of you!' I did all the right preparations, went drug-free, and pushed for two hours. Then Max's head got stuck and his heartbeat became erratic enough to warrant a C-section. Quick and uneventful, Max was healthy and nursing in minutes and all I ever needed was a little ibuprofen. Though you can't assume every C-section will be so forgiving, I was lucky enough to be back on my feet and walking again in days.

"Two years later, I pushed out Skye 'naturally' (although the casualness of that term never ceases to perplex me) and the whole bottom of my body was blown out. She wasn't even that big; 8 pounds, 2 ounces. But I couldn't walk normally for weeks. Visiting the bathroom was a lengthy, dreaded event. Nothing came out the way it was supposed to, and then it hurt. Healing from a C-section had been so easy and fast; now, two weeks after a 'normal' birth, I could only walk at a snail's pace, careful not to create any further disturbance. Sitting down was even worse. I was devastated.

"After four weeks I was finally feeling like my organs weren't going to drop out of my body when I walked, but things didn't completely heal until well into the second month. Although it took me months to get up the courage to really pick up my pace, let alone run anywhere there wasn't a bathroom, with long walks, basic abdominal work and many Kegels, I found myself pretty much back to normal. So even if you didn't have triplets or major surgery when you gave birth, it still might take a while to get your body back to feeling normal. Don't get discouraged . . . it's literally one step at a time.

— Lisa

- Eat properly and drink at least eight glasses of fluid a day (more if you're thirsty). This is especially important if you're nursing.

- Easy walking is fine, but get your doctor's okay or wait until you see your practitioner at the postpartum checkup (about six weeks) before you pick up the pace or start other more intense aerobic exercise.

Exercise After Cesarean Section

Though a delivery by C-section can seem to throw a wrench in the works, especially if it was unscheduled and unplanned, there's no reason that it has to undermine your postpartum recovery or even return to exercise. You'll no doubt be told by the physician that it was major surgery, and reminded of this by your body. You'll get clear instructions on caring for the incision, antibiotics and follow-up as determined by your doctor, and guidelines on how much you can do, and when. But there's no reason to presume you'll be relegated to bed or even prohibited from exercise.

Most doctors recognize that you're going to want to—and have to—get moving again as soon as possible with the new baby in the house. In fact, the Canadian Society for Exercise Physiology's guidelines are as clear as any on the topic: "Women who have had Caesarean delivery may slowly increase their aerobic and strength training, depending on their level of discomfort and other complicating factors such as anemia or wound infection." Up until the six-week postpartum doctor visit, your activity will generally be restricted to care of the baby and easy walking. But after that, a gradual return to your full exercise routine is likely. It's important to remember to avoid any movements or positions that cause stress or stretching across your stomach. Stay away from any increases in intra-abdominal pressure, such as twisting, pushing, or lifting something heavy or abruptly.

Coping with C-Section

Samantha Weld, 34, Medford, Massachusetts

After her son, Tommy, arrived by C-section, Samantha, right, was taking short walks as soon as she got home from the hospital. "I think my recovery was trouble-free because I was fit throughout my pregnancy, and because I got out right away afterward," she says. With her doc's okay and orders to start off slowly and avoid pushing and lifting, Sam was able to start walking right away. Her mother, who stayed with new parents Sam and husband Karl for a week after Tommy's arrival, pushed Tommy's carriage up the big hill they live on. Then Sam would push him on the flat sections. They turned back after five minutes, but it was a start that she gradually built on.

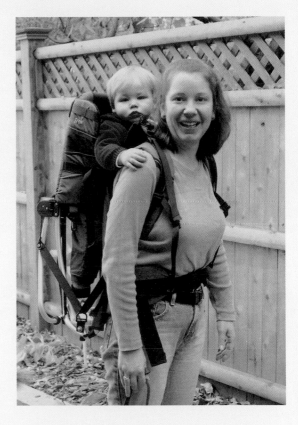

Sam was frustrated at first, because she wanted to do more. "The section wasn't planned, and since I walked through my whole pregnancy, I had thought I'd be able to jump back a lot more quickly." It took a month to feel comfortable with Tommy in the front carrier, and to be able to push the stroller with ease.

But her progress was steady and unmistakable, and her patience paid off. By the time Tommy was three months old, Sam was walking every day for at least 35 minutes around her suburban neighborhood with Tommy in a carriage or front carrier. By the time he reached 13 months, they kept up the same routine with a jogging stroller, and sometimes explored the trails in a nearby park. Most days, Sam walks with her neighbor and her toddler, getting the added benefit of social time. A few times a week, she gets in extra walking by running errands and going to the library and park on foot.

Walking is the cornerstone to a healthy lifestyle for Sam. "If I don't walk, I feel badly about myself, and then the snowball starts rolling. My downfall is cheese, and I'll start nibbling. And instead of cooking a healthy dinner, I'll order a loaded pizza or fried mozarrella sticks." But by walking regularly, she's more motivated to eat healthy foods, too. That, and the addition of working with free weights and a stability ball on alternate days, helped Sam lose the pregnancy weight and an additional 24 pounds—an impressive feat—by Tommy's first birthday.

When stretching, hold each position for 30 seconds, relaxing and breathing deeply. Feel only a gentle pull; never stretch to the point of discomfort.

Nursing and Exercise: A Perfect Combination

There's no reason that a healthy nursing mom can't also be an active mom. You might have heard that babies refuse to nurse from mothers who have just exercised, because lactic acid released during physical exertion alters the taste of their milk. The latest data shows that this is not a concern with moderate levels of exercise. Unless you're doing sprints until you collapse or logging marathon-type mileage, baby should accept milk happily, even right on the heels of a workout.

Nursing moms also may worry that exercise may change the quantity or quality of their milk, putting baby at risk for slow growth. But fear not, because studies have shown that moderate exercise won't cause any of these problems, and that it's safe for both baby and Mom.

More at issue: Both exercise and lactation take energy. That's already in high demand for new mothers who have disrupted sleep and are dealing with physical and emotional stress. But it's excessive fatigue, *not* exercise per se, that will challenge successful breast-feeding. This means nursing moms need to pay extra attention to getting more (or at least better) sleep–which can be aided by exercise– what they drink, and making sure they get up to 200 more calories a day than they did while pregnant.

An additional concern raised by researchers is whether exercise alters the immunity levels in breast milk. Though very vigorous exercise seems to be linked to lower immunity levels in a mother's milk, the milk returns to a normal level within an hour of the workout. And again, this only in the case of really hard exercise–a sustained dose of power lifting or a very long run–which is not an issue for most moms, especially in the first months postpartum. If you do plan to really get back into serious training, simply allow for your body to recover for an hour after hard workouts before breast-feeding.

THE BENEFITS OF BREAST-FEEDING

Given that there's no downside to nursing and exercise, let's think about why it's so beneficial to both you and the baby to breast-feed as long as possible. After all, this is a health book, and there are plenty of health benefits. Babies who are breast-fed have been shown to suffer fewer colds and infections, reflecting the stronger immune capacity passed on from Mom. Breast-fed babies also show the healthiest growth rates, and even improved learning (though this may be related to more nurturing settings, as well as the nursing itself). But equally important may be the benefits to mothers. Women who breast-feed are at markedly reduced risk for breast cancer later in life, and they show a reduced risk for obesity. Researchers suspect the calories burned producing milk for the baby help mothers lose and keep off excess weight in the critical postpartum period, although some breast-feeding moms find it hard to lose those last few pounds until they've weaned.

To keep yourself comfortable and baby optimally fed, follow these guidelines:
▪Drink up. You need a minimum of eight glasses of fluid a day (preferably water), but many nursing moms feel so thirsty all the time that they drink like camels, and easily down much more.

Walking and Nursing Worked

Samantha Weld

"Exercising and nursing was no big deal for me. Most important, get a good sports bra and be aware that you'll need to drink a lot of water. I occasionally brought a bottle with me, but most often I just made sure to drink plenty before and after. I didn't bother to buy a special nursing sports bra because who wants to nurse your baby closely in a stinky sweaty bra? At first I just put a sports bra over my nursing bra. And later, I just wore a regular sports bra. Support is the key! As for timing, I went walking after nursing, because I didn't want Tommy to be hungry while I was trying to walk and have that cut it short."

▪ Fuel up. Small, frequent meals and substantial but nutritious snacks (see chapter 13) will give you the energy to walk and produce plenty of milk. Women who aren't pregnant or nursing need 1,800 to 2,200 calories a day. If you're at a healthy weight (not overweight), you may need up to 500 more while you're nursing.

▪ Stick to regular but moderate levels of exercise to avoid getting overtired.

▪ Nurse before you walk or work out. Two big benefits: One, you're much more likely to complete your workout without having to stop to nurse. Two, you'll be that much more comfortable.

▪ Wear a supportive, breathable bra that supports you during exercise. Tender, enlarged breasts and a flimsy bra add up to lots of discomfort. Though they're not cheap, consider it money well spent to buy a bra that will keep you comfortable enough to keep walking.

▪ Talk to your doctor about whether you should be taking a vitamin supplement. One recent study showed that vitamin B_6 levels, as well as infant growth rates, were the same for breast-feeding mothers who exercised and moderately reduced their calorie intake as they were for nonexercising moms, as long as the exercisers took a vitamin supplement and ate a nutritionally balanced diet.

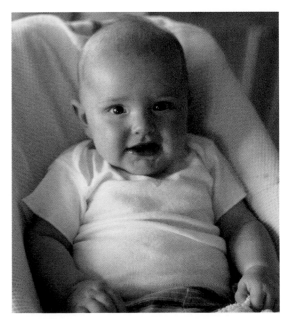

Down but Not Out: Routine Blues and Postpartum Depression

It's common for new mothers to experience a down-and-out sort of feeling that's often called the baby blues. When you consider all you're dealing with—a major life event, new responsibility, fatigue, dropping hormone levels—it's not surprising that 70 percent of all new moms go through this phase, marked by feeling fragile and experiencing stress, anxiety, sadness, and anger. This may last a couple of hours, or hang around for a week or two. What makes it all worse is that after nine months of building expectations, you think you *ought* to feel like you're on top of the world.

HERE ARE FIVE WAYS TO HELP COPE:

1. Rest. Crash early. Nap when baby naps. Forget the housework and put your feet up.
2. Don't isolate yourself. Talk with your partner, your mom, dad, sister, aunt, cousin, or a friend about what you're feeling. A sister or girlfriend who's been through this may help you see that yes, it's normal. Joining a new mother's group where you can hear that other new moms are treading the same path can also help.
3. Learn to say yes. To every offer for help, that is. You don't have to be superwoman. Take your friends up on arranging to cook dinner for a week. Let your neighbor pick up the milk or walk the dog or watch your toddler for an hour. If you need extra hands, consider hiring help, even just short term. The payoff—your peace of mind—is well worth it.
4. In two-parent households, think and talk openly about the division of labor—there's plenty to go around. Though you may think you have to do everything, you may well have a partner who would cherish more time with the baby but doesn't feel able to intrude on your mother-child experience.
5. And of course, take at least a short walk every day. Exercise, a proven mood lifter, can also prevent postpartum depression, provided it doesn't create stress for you. No matter how short your time, get out and walk.

GOOD QUESTION

How do I know if I'm really depressed, or just tired?

The American Council of Obstetricians and Gynecologists offers the following warning signs that your blues may be a more serious clinical depression. If you experience any of these, talk to your doctor right away:

- Feelings of sadness that persist for more than two weeks after baby's birth.
- Experiencing depression or anger four to eight weeks after baby's birth.
- Sadness, hopelessness, guilt, worry, or doubt that persist, get progressively worse, or interfere with daily life.
- Over- or undereating.
- Excessive sleeping, even when baby is awake.
- Insomnia—the inability to sleep even when the baby is.
- Overwhelming worry about or disinterest in your baby.
- Thoughts of harming yourself or your baby.
- Panic attacks.

Bottom Line: If you're feeling persistent blues, anger, worry, or sadness, or any dangerous feelings toward yourself or the baby, then you must seek help right away. Having a new baby is an extraordinary challenge, and it's not a sign of weakness to feel overwhelmed; it's even possible that biochemical or hormonal changes are at the root of your feelings. But you have to take action and get help for any of it to get better.

If the blues intensify or last longer, you might be dealing with a more serious condition, postpartum depression. In that case, get help right away. Call your ob-gyn, who can help set up treatment and counseling.

Taking Baby Out

Amid the challenges of learning to nurse or give bottles, change diapers, and otherwise cope on very little sleep, you will reach a point where fresh air and motion sound like a good thing. Don't push yourself to try for serious exercise before you feel up to it, but once you do, trust that it's good for baby, too. And if you plan on physical activity becoming a routine part of your life with the baby—and you should—then it's best to establish the habit early.

Although one approach would be to get babysitters or have someone else in the household watch the baby while you go and exercise, the fact is that you're better off figuring out how to be active *with* your child right from the beginning. This means you won't be dependent on others for your chances to walk. Instead, you'll be a self-reliant exercise team.

Relax—though babies seem fragile, there's no reason to shut them up inside. "For one, germs have a lot less chance of living outside than in a stuffy house," says William Boyle, MD, a pediatrician at The Children's Hospital at Dartmouth in Lebanon, New Hampshire, and a fellow of the American Academy of Pediatrics. "If you're active and you like to be outside, you don't have to stay in." Plus, there's myriad equipment and clothing available to keep babies safe and cozy while you go break a sweat. For a detailed summary of the gear for taking baby along on a walk, see chapter 11; each piece will then be detailed at the appropriate postmester: front carriers and strollers in chapter 11, jogging strollers in chapter 14, baby backpacks in chapter 17.

BE A SMART WALKING TEAM

When you and baby start walking together, you may find it takes time to iron out some of the details. When you walked alone or with friends, there wasn't much chance that someone might get angry if she dropped her Binky or filled a diaper.

Take It from Us:

Breast-feeding may be the best feeding for active travel.

Breast-feeding a baby doesn't mean your travels are restricted to the mailbox and back. Mark and I traveled to Mount Washington for a friend's wedding, and it was clear early on there was no way we were going to be that close to the wilderness and not do some hiking. But this mountain is no place for two little ones (ages three years and six months at the time), and I was still breast-feeding daughter Skye, so didn't want to leave her at home. We booked a suite near a playground and an indoor swimming pool. And in addition to Gramma and Grampa in tow, these key essentials made it possible to have an incredible, all-day adventure. Oh, and the wedding was fun, too.

"My recommended traveler's nursing kit includes :

- "A mini electric (Medela) or hand (Avent) breast pump.
- "Medela CSF Milk Bags let you collect, store, and freeze your milk in the same bag. They're self-closing, leakproof, and sterile.
- "Soothies gel breast pads provide natural moisture, prevent bacterial growth, and won't stick to skin. They're great for preventing chafing on a long hike.
- "A Medela small cooler/carrier has two separate compartments—one for a small pump, the other insulated to carry milk—and a small ice pack.

"And all of this is small enough to fit handily in (Mark's) backpack!

—*Lisa*

Nor did loading a surprisingly agile little one into the front carrier double the time it took you to get out the door. But you'll find you both get the routine down pretty quickly—and you'll both do better if you make it a regular habit, not a once-in-a-while adventure. Here are some tips for those first walks.

- **Take a trial run.** If you decide to use a front carrier, practice putting it on several times without baby to get the hang of it, and to get the adjustments as close as you can to a good fit (you'll have to tweak things once baby's on board). Don't panic if the first few times those squirmy little legs just don't seem to want to go in right. It's not a bad idea to have an extra person around in case you need a hand the first few times you mount up; don't worry, you'll both quickly get the hang of it.

- **Watch your footing.** Slippery conditions are double trouble if you're carrying or pushing

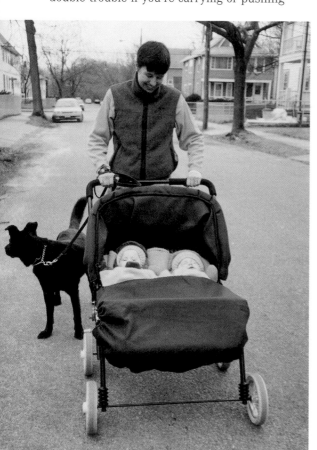

baby. Avoid ice, hard-packed snow, mud, and anything else that looks slick if you've got baby in a front carrier or in the stroller. Because you're not in your usual physical shape after delivery, you're less likely to be able to catch yourself if you slip or lose your balance, and a fall could injure baby or send the stroller flying.

- **Leave the bottle at home.** Don't get into the habit of popping a bottle into baby's mouth when you pop him into the stroller. "Babies who always suck bottles as they fall asleep are prone to milk caries or cavities from the milk that remains in their mouth," explains Ann Hansen, MD, a neonatologist at the Children's Hospital in Boston. Plus, it can end up frustrating the baby if a jostling ride causes him to lose the bottle.

- **Think like a baby.** Okay, at first this will seem hopeless. Why is she crying on the walk today, but yesterday—when everything was identical—she slept like a, well, you know? Consider the obvious stuff, of course—when she last ate or got a clean diaper. But also try to *be* her. Are there any straps or harnesses pinching where you can't see? Have you just turned the stroller so that the warm sun you're so enjoying is right in her eyes? Did a hat slip down over her face, or the wind shift? With time, you'll get to understand every squeak and giggle.

WHAT ABOUT THE WEATHER?

It's easier than you think for a baby to be able to join you on a walk in almost any weather—even when you find it warmer or colder than comfortable. The baby's not exercising and generating body heat, he's just along for the ride. So on warm days, with proper protection from the sun, comfortable clothes, and the movement of air from your walk, he can be quite comfortable even as you're drenched in sweat. On cold days, you can provide the baby protection from the wind and chill, safely cocooning her in her stroller or carrier, or tucking her front carrier in close under your coat to benefit from your body heat. In either case, we've found that our babies were

Making It All Fit In

Allison Librett, 34, Atlanta, Georgia

As a mother of two (Sophie, 3, and Nicholas, 1), part-time lawyer, and occasional fitness instructor, Allison is used to having to work hard to fit it all in. Despite juggling all the balls that many moms have to keep in the air—child care, housekeeping, part-time work—she's proof that making physical activity a priority can actually help. In fact, she's the first to tell you that exercise is one key to keeping everything running smoothly. "Exercising, either with the kids or without, makes me feel more in control of my life," she says. "It gives me energy, and helps control stress. If I don't exercise, I'm less tolerant of the numerous questions and demands of everyday life. With exercise, I'm able to be more focused and enjoy being a kid with my two little ones."

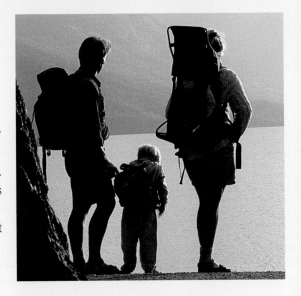

Staying flexible about activities has been a big factor in helping Allison find time to exercise. Over the years, she's done everything from walk with her baby in the backpack to teaching aerobics to doing yoga with her toddler. Flexing the schedule helps, too. On some days, an early-morning swim before the kids wake is ideal; on others, nap times are a better bet.

Allison's Five Ways for Mom to Fit in Fitness

■ **SET UP A HOME GYM.** It doesn't have to be elaborate or pricey, but with the right gear a home gym is open anytime you're free, and there's never a commute. Allison and her husband stocked their house with free weights in 5-, 10-, 15-, and 20-pound increments, along with a medicine ball, elastic exercise bands, a yoga mat, and a bike stand that converts her bike to a stationary cycle right on the porch.

■ **TAKE ADVANTAGE OF NAP TIME.** When Sophie naps in the afternoon, Allison lifts weights or pedals the bike. If Nicholas is up, he watches from nearby.

■ **BUILD IT INTO THE SCHEDULE.** Allison cemented her commitment to working out by becoming an instructor, though not everyone can teach a Spinning class twice a week, as she has. But committing to leading exercise walks for the YMCA, nature walks for the school, or helping maintain a community garden could build *scheduled* activity into your week. "I can't cancel, and I know I'll get at least two hours of exercise a week," she says. And regarding an exercise class: "If I wanted to be there anyway, I might as well get paid for it."

■ **LOOK AT IT AS A BREAK.** "Going off to exercise by myself is a real treat," she says. "For one hour, I don't have to keep track of what Sophie might be doing to Nicholas, or whether Nick needs to be fed."

■ **TRADE TIME WITH YOUR HUSBAND.** Allison's husband works out, too, so they work together and swap parenting duties to get their workouts in.

■ **TAKE THE KID(S) ALONG.** Front carriers, double strollers, and backpacks provide all the hardware you need to take them along when that's the best option.

Record the time of day you walk. Do you walk farther or faster in the morning, or are your best walks in the evening?

often far more comfortable than we were when out in inclement weather. Here are some specific tips for getting out for a walk any time of year:

- **Heat health.** Until the age of six months, the best way to shield baby from the sun's harmful rays is with clothing or full shade. Use the stroller or pram hood to block sun; even some baby backpacks (for older babies) have sun screens and hoods. Dress baby in a brimmed bonnet and keep skin covered as much as you can without causing baby to overheat. Stick to shady areas, and choose early- or late-day outings when the sun's rays are less direct. Go with loose-fitting (except for the diaper, of course), airy, light-colored clothing. Also, try to arrange the stroller so that even as the sun is blocked, air can flow through while you walk and induce a slight breeze.

- **Cold comfort.** "It's never too cold to go out, as long as you're comfortable and baby is dressed appropriately," says Dr. Boyle. Start off with a dry diaper; dryness equals warmth. Dress baby in layers, ending with a warm bunting and a snug hat to avoid losing that 25 to 30 percent of heat that escapes from his head. Apply a thin layer of petroleum jelly (for example, Vaseline) to keep face and lips from chapping; this especially helps with babies who drool a lot.

Take It from Us:

The baby can handle whatever you can handle.

"My first winter with Natalie (my third child, after twins) was one of the coldest on the Maine books. For weeks the thermometer seemed stuck between 0 and 15 degrees Fahrenheit. (We knew it was bad when 20 degrees felt balmy, and 30 plus sun provoked a family picnic in the backyard on just-made snow benches.) Still, I bundled up Natalie and trudged out for a walk on most days, with our Lab Trapper in tow.

"She was about two months old when the first snow hit. To keep her warm, I tucked her in a fleecy suit and hat, put her in the Baby Björn front carrier, and then zipped Matt's parka over both of us, leaving the top open so she could get fresh air. She never complained a bit, and usually fell promptly asleep.

"My other option was a great pram that I bought second- (or maybe third-) hand through the paper. Its big wheels and suspension made for a smooth ride, and the bassinet and hood kept Natalie well out of the wind. When she was a little past five months old, I was able to put her safely in the jogging stroller. Especially on frigid days, she was always well bundled (regular outfit plus a

fleece suit, topped with a hat and zipped into a wonderful sleeping-bag-like sack with legs), and the wind cover on the jogger was a must to protect her from arctic air. Footing was sometimes a challenge. You never knew when you'd get ice, slush, or even a section of snow-covered road. Sneakers were deadly. I opted for hiking boots or insulated winter snow boots, and though they slowed me down, the traction and warmth were well worth it.

"We had our daily walking date in the early afternoon, when the sun and the temperature were as high as they would get, and while the big sisters were off at kindergarten. Though we didn't rack up big mileage, even 20 or 30 minutes did wonders for my spirit. I got a lift from the fresh air and motion, and tried to focus on the sun sparkling on new snow, or icicles jangling on the bushes in the wind, instead of my freezing ears. I know my neighbors probably thought I was nuts. Some people are just better off on a treadmill inside while their baby naps. But for me, getting outdoors in winter—even in the bitter cold—was the only way to survive it.

— *Tracy*

Depending on the temperature, you might need to do one or all of these: Line the pram or stroller with a blanket before you put baby in, tuck another blanket over and around baby, attach a rain cover to block the wind and keep warmth in. Don't neglect sun protection even in winter. It's especially important if there's snow on the ground, which can reflect harmful rays.

If you're using a front carrier, your body will help warm baby, too. Tucking a blanket around the outside of the carrier and zipping your coat around it can provide another warm layer in cold conditions. Just use extra caution with newborns. "For young babies with questionable neck and head control, the worst thing you can do is bundle them up to the point where you can't see them breathing or see the color of their skin," warns Dr. Hansen. A mother who has walked with all three of her children in carriers as infants in cold weather, Hansen frequently checked for proper breathing by placing her hand a few inches from baby's mouth and nose. "You don't have to stare at them, but do keep checking," she says.

GOALS ARE GREAT, BUT MAY NOT BE ENOUGH

No doubt you've heard that setting goals is critical for making an exercise habit stick. But a recent study shows that how you implement the goal is just as important as setting it. Danielle Symons Downs, PhD, from the Pennsylvania State University and Robert Singer, PhD, from the University of Florida divided male and female college students into two groups. Both groups were tested for performance on one-minute push-up and curl-up tests, and scheduled for a retest eight weeks later. One group was told how to set goals; the second was given detailed information on how to implement their goals by planning where, when, and how to pursue them. While both groups received feedback on goal setting, the second group also got a weekly reminder to plan and organize their exercise time. As the researchers

anticipated, the group that learned how, when, and where to implement their plans outperformed the group that simply set goals.

For busy mothers who are tackling new and probably unfamiliar responsibilities at the same time that they also may hope to stay active and shed the weight they gained during their pregnancy, this takes on special importance.

The key is to arm yourself with the tools (the how, what, why, when) to meet your exercise goals successfully. "For example, if I want to lose 5 pounds, I need a plan," says Downs. "I have to specify when I will do this by providing a time frame (by November 30). I want to think about how I will do this (drink one less soda at 250 calories a day for a total savings of 1,750 calories a week, and increase my walks by 10 minutes three times a week to burn more calories), and where I will do this (say, walk at home; have one less soda at work)."

You'll be even more likely to succeed if you build in time each week to plan the specifics for the week ahead. Set aside a specific time, maybe Sunday morning after breakfast, and sit down with your calendar. Block out the time you need for exercise (which days? nap time? early morning? early evening?), exactly what you're going to do, for how long, and where you're going to do it, and make any arrangements for child care that need to happen. "Anyone can set goals, but accomplishing them takes proper planning, preparation, and organizational skills that often take time to practice," adds Downs. That means this is the perfect time to get into the habit of using an exercise log like the one described in this book, if you haven't already. But don't just record your exercise after the fact. Follow Dr. Downs's advice and actually think a week or two ahead, jotting down some specifics—whom you're meeting to walk and when, or which day you plan to do a longer walk—right in the diary to act as a reminder and motivator.

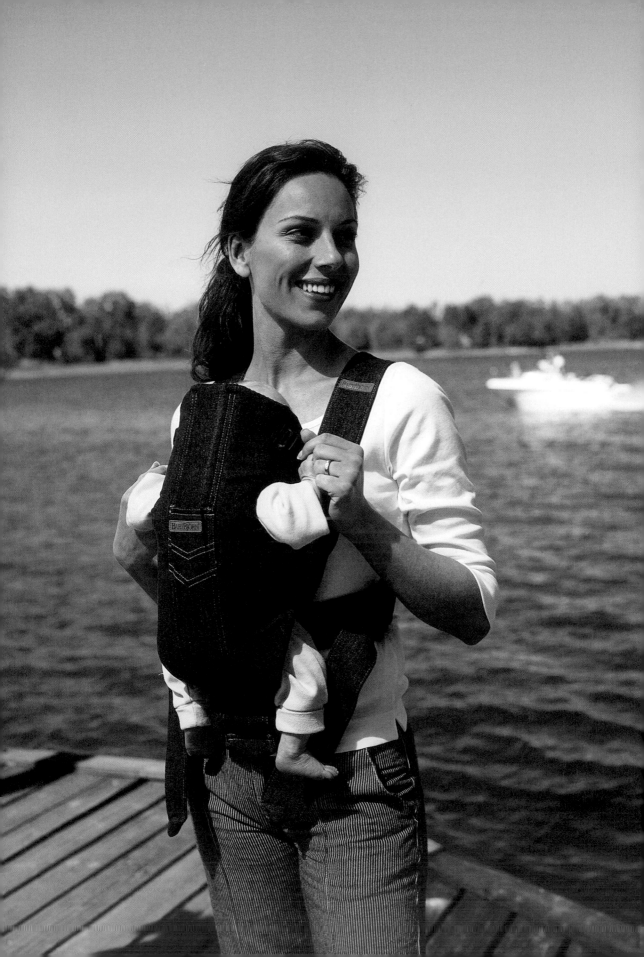

Gear 404: Getting Baby Out the Door

You and Baby: An Exercise Team

No doubt one approach to postpartum exercise is swapping child-care duties with a spouse or friend and heading out to walk alone. But there are plenty of reasons to bring the baby along. You and your child both need time outdoors in natural light and fresh air, plus it gives you the flexibility to go when and for however long you want, not just when a sitter's available. You'll also be introducing your child to being active every day right from the beginning—a gift that we've all seen manifest in the active lives of our young children already.

If baby's coming along for a walk, you want to make sure you're using a carrier or stroller that matches your child's physical development. At very least, if a baby is flopping around uncomfortably on a walk you can be sure it's the last thing she'll be interested in the next time around. But far worse, an infant can be badly hurt if she ends up in an awkward position that pinches a limb or impedes her breathing. So read carefully this summary of the hardware that's available to take the baby along as she gains greater and greater control. Each is described in more detail, along with buying and use tips, at the appropriate gear chapter over the four postmesters of the book. Front carriers and regular strollers are detailed later in this chapter; jogging strollers are in chapter 14, baby backpacks in chapter 17, and bicycle seats and trailers are in chapter 20.

How to Start Out

Front carriers, pram-style carriages, strollers that have a bassinet conversion or can be fitted with an infant car seat, or wheeled frames to which you can attach an infant car seat may all be fitting choices for your newborn's early outings. It's essential to check the manufacturer's instructions for each specific piece of equipment, because the guidelines for appropriate age, length, and weight vary from product to product.

For newborns, the biggest issue is supporting baby's wobbly head and neck. Until he's strong enough to gain some control, his head and neck need constant support or there is a risk of obstructing his airway. Premature babies, babies with low muscle tone or strength, or babies who are small for their gestational age are most at risk. If your baby was born at 37 weeks or earlier, the hospital staff may perform a car seat test to make sure baby can safely ride in a car seat without concern that his head and neck would collapse forward or sideways and obstruct his airway. "Babies who pass this should be okay in a carrier that positions baby

Get a front carrier *now.*

Our front carriers were a godsend with fussy, colicky twins. In the early weeks, my husband and I used to each load up a baby at night and circle the block until they settled down. With our third, the carrier kept my hands free for some critical time each afternoon, saving us from ordering pizza every night. Plus, it enabled me to get outside to play hide-and-seek with our older girls with the peace of mind that the baby was close, safe, and content.

—Tracy

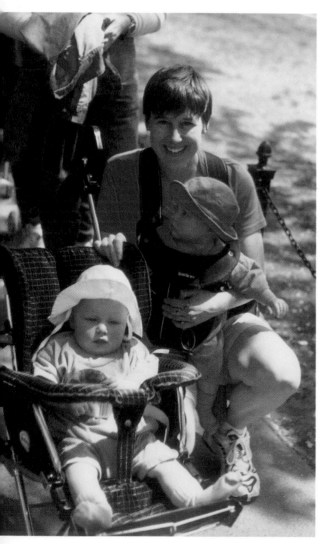

somewhat upright, provided their head and neck are well supported," says Dr. Hansen of Boston's Children's Hospital.

PRAMS, BASSINETS, STROLLERS

Bassinet-style prams and strollers that recline flat and are designed for young babies are safest for newborns, provided they are placed on their backs. (The same safe-sleep guidelines apply to carriages as the crib: Baby should lie on her back, with no loose blankets or toys that could offer a choking hazard.) This is the safest position for young babies who don't have the head and neck control to recover if they slump or tilt to the side or front, which are positions that can cause the airway to kink and block. Some units allow you to put the car seat on board—use the same care in setting the angle of incline as you do placing it in the car.

INCLINED CARRIAGE SEATS

You'll know baby is ready to ride in an inclined position when he can lift his head off the mattress. "Then he's strong and coordinated enough to be in other positions," says Hansen. At this point, a 30- to 40-degree angle is most comfortable. Double-check that baby doesn't slump forward or sideways or fold at the middle when seated in a reclined position in the stroller or stroller-mounted car seat.

FRONT CARRIERS—FACING YOU

"Babies gain some head and neck control between two and three months of age, so if you use a carrier before that, it must support baby's head and keep her from slumping," says JoAnn Rohyans, MD, a spokesperson for the American Academy of Pediatrics and a member of the pediatric department at the Ohio State University College of Medicine in Columbus. "The chin should not hit the chest." So the baby will start in a front carrier riding facing you, with her head completely supported. Some carriers set a minimum weight recommendation of 8 pounds.

FRONT CARRIERS—FACING THE WORLD

When baby gains some degree of head control, he may soon reach another turning point. "For a long time babies love to gaze into their parents' faces for comfort. Then the fascination ends, and they want to see dogs and trees and houses and cars," says Hansen. If your front carrier is designed to let baby ride facing both ways, this is a good point to try turning baby around so he can see the world. "If baby has the head control, take cues from how he acts at home," says Hansen. If he is fussy or seems bored, and if he's spending less time staring at you and more scoping out the room, try turning him around in the carrier; some carriers have a recommended age for this. But because of widely differing development rates, rely on your judgment and that of your pediatrician.

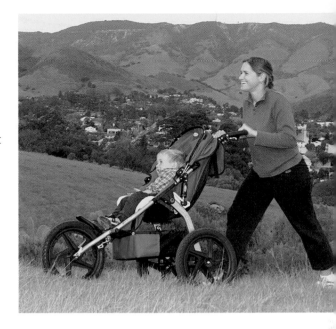

"JOGGING" STROLLERS

Jogging strollers have three air-filled tires—one in front, two in the rear—and a fabric seat slung within its lightweight frame. Though best for an infant with a strong torso and neck and total head control (usually over five months), some "jogger" manufacturers have designed infant inserts to make their strollers safe for babies at about two months of age. (Generally, the fabric seats alone have too little support and too much room for newborns.) Don't assume a jogger stroller with an insert is okay just because your baby meets the age and weight guidelines. First try this test: Place baby on a blanket on her tummy. If she lifts her head up off the floor and turns it to the side, she has some degree of head and neck control, and you may be good to go. If her nose stays on the floor (not surprisingly, a cause for tears), she's not ready yet.

But still make this final check: Strap baby into the jogger with the insert, and push the stroller gently over a bump as you watch. "If she slides from side to side and can't keep her neck straight, or if her head falls forward or to either side, she's not ready yet," says Hansen. If you use your jogger with an insert, remember that speed and bumps are especially jarring for young babies

who can't control their bodies. Stick with walking and stay on smooth terrain, such as sidewalks and pavement. And because jogging strollers position baby away from you, opt for one with a peekaboo window in the hood that allows you to make sure a young baby remains safely upright.

READINESS RECAP: SAFE GEAR FOR BABY'S EARLY OUTINGS

Hopefully, we're convincing you that with proper clothing and gear, a baby will enjoy and even thrive outdoors with you in just about any conditions. So here's a quick recap of the hardware available, from the front carriers and various strollers detailed in this chapter to further gear that's described in later chapters, when appropriate for baby.

Flat Strollers and Prams or Bassinet-Style Carriages

- Safe for newborns, provided you follow the same safety rules as when you put them down in bed—they ride on their backs, nothing to get tangled in or covering their mouth, and so forth.

Reclining Strollers

- Safe when baby can lift his head off the mattress.
- Use at a 30- to 40-degree angle.

Front Carriers

- Follow manufacturer's guidelines for age, weight, and length.
- The carrier must hold baby upright with head and neck support so her chin does not hit her chest (this is a concern until baby can lift her head off a mattress, generally between two and three months).
- Premature or underweight babies should also pass the hospital car seat test before using carriers.

Jogging Strollers with Infant Inserts

- For complete details, see chapter 14.
- Follow the manufacturer's guidelines for age and weight.
- These are safe when baby can lift his head off the floor or mattress and turn it to the side, at approximately two to three months.
- Make sure baby rides upright with a straight neck, and doesn't flop sideways or forward.
- To use without an insert, wait until baby has full trunk, head, and neck control, usually at around six months.

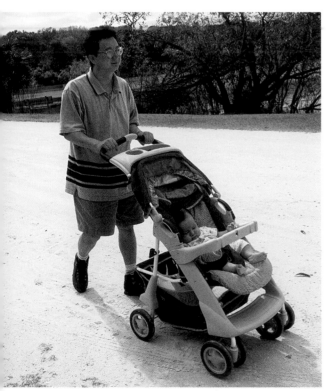

Backpacks

- For complete details, see chapter 17.
- Follow manufacturer's guidelines for age and weight, and try it out for fit.
- Backpacks are *not* appropriate for early outings; they're safe only when baby has full neck strength and head control—likely over five months for most babies.
- Try out both entry and exit, and how it carries, to be sure it works for both baby and you.

Buying a Front Carrier

Once you try a soft front carrier, you'll see that those canny kangaroos are on to something. Made from a cloth pouch for baby and an attached harness that supports baby's weight and goes over your shoulders, soft carriers are designed to keep baby close to your chest. Babies favor this proximity to Mom, but it's also great because sometimes Mom needs both hands free. Carriers give you the best of both worlds, snuggling baby while giving you some freedom to go for a walk, run errands, or just get chores done around the house.

Beyond a way to get you moving, you'll quickly find that a sturdy carrier is worth its weight in gold for those times when you can't both comfort baby and keep life running smoothly. The witching hours of late afternoon and evening, when most babies get fussy and of course you're often trying to get a meal on the table, can be prime carrier time. Most carriers are for babies who weigh 8 or more pounds (check the manufacturer's guidelines).

Cost: $20-$120, with most over $50.

Upside: Frees your hands and gives mobility while keeping baby close. Most are designed so that as babies get older, they can turn from facing you to facing outward for a better view.

Downside: Relatively short window of service, especially for bigger babies, because most get too heavy to be carried this way before they reach the carrier's upper weight limit (roughly 30 pounds). Some are complicated to use, so make sure you try them on at a store before you make a purchase. They may cause sore shoulders or neck for parents, so build up gradually.

Look for these features for baby:

- Plenty of head and neck support for young babies, who don't have control of their upper bodies.
- A position that holds baby upright without putting all her weight on her bottom to protect the spine and lower back.
- Support under the backs of the legs, in a position where the knees are lower than the buttocks.
- Leg openings that won't let baby slip through.
- Adjustments that let the carrier grow with baby.
- Reversability, so baby can ride facing you and later, facing out.
- Sturdy fabric and hardware.

Look for these features for you:

- Ease of adjustment and loading/unloading. Putting the carrier on should be quick, and you shouldn't need a helper to get baby safely in and out.
- Wide, padded straps that distribute baby's weight evenly and comfortably.
- Adjustments that let you position baby comfortably and that allow another adult to fit the carrier to his or her body.
- Machine washable.

Nice extras: Lumbar support is a plus for active parents who will wear the carrier for longer stretches of time.

Brands include: Baby Björn, Snugli (Evenflo), Kelty, Maclaren, Infantino, Walking Rock Farm (which offers the Hip Baby, a great product for older babies but designed more for around the house and errands than actual exercise walking).

Picking Out Some Wheels— Strollers

A good set of wheels may be a mom's best friend, and we don't mean the motorized kind. Equipping yourself with a sturdy stroller or two is one of the best investments you can make if you want to stay active as a parent. Strollers keep baby safe and comfortable, and, soothed by motion, most happily snooze as they roll. As your child gets older and is more plugged into her surroundings, she'll find

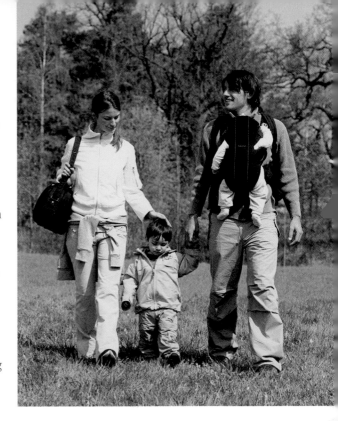

watching the scenery change and learning about the world 50 times better than *Teletubbies*. What's in it for you? A chance to rest your arms and back, get fresh air and exercise, and also run errands and walk the dog, all with a happy baby.

Though you may need no convincing on the beauty of strollers, deciding which one to buy is another story. Indeed, visit any baby store or surf the Internet for strollers and the options can make you dizzy in minutes. To help you sort out what you need, we'll walk through the field, outlining each type and its strengths and weaknesses. Keep in mind that many parents don't find one ideal stroller to fit all their needs, and often end up buying two or more.

PRAMS

You may feel like an English nanny at the helm, but these traditional carriages—like bassinets on wheels—have a wonderful gliding ride for newborns and young babies. Many are designed so the bassinet can be removed or converted to a standard stroller for older babies. Some have adjustable handlebars and can be set up so baby can ride facing or away from you. If cost is an obstacle, consider borrowing one or buying a used pram for the early months.

Cost: $250–$575.

Upside: Newborns can ride in them right away. Durable and strong. Big, rubber wheels and suspension create an extremely smooth ride for baby. Fixed wheels track well for fast walking but may be awkward for negotiating lots of turns. Hood and high sides protect baby from weather. Removable bassinets can double for use in the house.

Downside: Heavy and cumbersome to transport. Fast or long-legged walkers may kick the frame. Pricey.

Make sure: You have room to store a carriage of this size. If you don't live on the ground floor, getting it up and down stairs is a challenge.

Nice extras: An apron or boot that covers the bassinet for extra warmth and wind protection. Mosquito netting.

Brands include: Emmaljunga, Bertini, Britax, Inglesina, Peg Perego, Chicco, Silver Cross.

STANDARD STROLLERS

These are the basic workhorses you see all over every mall in America. They're popular because they accommodate babies from newborn through toddlerhood without breaking the bank, with features such as adjustable harnesses, multiple recline positions, and comfortable, padded interiors. Wheels are typically hard plastic, and the front wheels can either swivel for easy maneuvering (in a store) or lock in place when you're walking a longer distance (to the park). Most have a roomy basket underneath for Mom to stash stuff. Less expensive models are made with more plastic and less metal, and are likely to be less durable in the long run.

For twins or families with two close in age, there are tandem models where one rides in front of the other (tricky to navigate on curbs), and side-by-side models (may not fit through all doorways). Still another option: An inexpensive simple stroller frame converts most infant car seats to a stroller by snapping the seat to the frame.

Take It from Us:

Taking baby out anytime.

"Don't let anyone tell you infants can't handle walking outside in winter. About six weeks after Maxwell was born, Lisa and I used a gift of a long-weekend stay we'd been given at the Trapp Family Lodge in Stowe, Vermont. The condo was cozy and the town delightful, and we spent a lot of time strolling the shops and walking along a beautiful multiuse trail down in the valley.

"The third day we were there a magnificent snow fell, covering the cross-country ski trails. Normally we'd have been out skiing (and falling) in a flash. But I'm realistic about my skill level—or lack thereof—and we were actually enjoying just relaxing without a telephone or the stream of visitors that had followed Max's arrival. So we decided on a moonlight walk along one of the ski trails with Max tucked into the front carrier and bundled in a head-to-toe fleece bunt with fold-over covers for his hands and feet, all zipped under my parka.

"Unfortunately, we forgot the trail map and flashlight, stumbled into deep snow, tried to take a 'shortcut' back to what turned out to be the wrong lights in the distance, and basically did all the things we 'experienced' hikers tell novices never to do, turning our 20-minute stroll into an icy hour-plus epic. The more we floundered, the more the wind howled!

"When we got back to the condo, we both admitted being really nervous that we'd had Max out too long in too cold conditions. But I was constantly checking him, and he'd slept contentedly while I was postholing up to my hips in new powder. He was none the worse for wear, despite rosy cheeks and ice crystals on the brim of his bunt.

"We don't recommend such a walk for everyone, but it's reassuring to know that if babies are kept warm and comfy and close, they're amazingly happy outdoors."

—Mark

GOOD QUESTION

How do I dress the baby for walking outside, especially in very cold or warm weather?

Use the same basic principles you would for yourself, keeping in mind that in winter the baby isn't generating any heat through exercise, and in summer his new skin is much more sensitive to the sun than yours. Always start with a dry diaper. In summer, go with a broad-brimmed hat or bonnet and light comfortable fabrics covering all exposed skin—unless you have a stroller with a full hood, your best bet to assure protection from the sun.

In winter, build layers for warmth. Use a thick fleece unit as the prime insulator. There are lots of one-piece units (bunts) to choose from. Most cover hands and feet—extra vulnerable in babies—and some are designed like a sack so both legs are together, for newborns. These can be very cozy, but can't be worn if you're using a front carrier—baby's legs pass through separate leg holes—or if you want to add another wind-resistant layer such as a one-piece snowsuit. Then tuck in a blanket around the stroller and use a wind hood, or zip the front carrier into your jacket, on the coldest days. Use a little petroleum jelly on any skin (cheeks, nose) that might be exposed to the biting wind.

Most important, check baby for comfort often. In warm weather, hydration is as important (or more)

for the baby as it is for you, so keep her well fed. (Signs of dehydration and overheating requiring immediate treatment include reduced urination, flushed dry skin, and a slight depression of the skin over the soft spot on the head.) In winter, watch for overheating—crying, flushed cheeks—as well as cold. Again the warnings are crying and cold fingertips, toes, and face—the first parts to suffer.

Bottom Line: The baby can handle anything you can, with the added advantage that he's not exercising, which heats you up in summer, and he can be given the extra protection (say, from wind or sun) of his stroller or carrier. Keep in mind that his skin is extra sensitive, and he's not moving and generating heat like you are. Focus on protection from the sun and wind, and you'll have a blast outside.

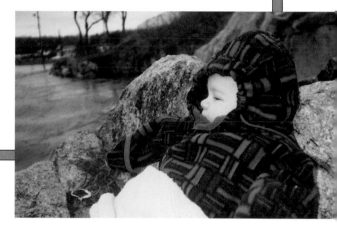

Best for errands and short walks.

Cost: $80-$300.

Upside: Long window of use with baby.

Downside: Too heavy and awkward for fitness walking.

Make sure: The stroller is easy to fold and stow if you want to take it in and out of the car often.

Nice extras: Some strollers are designed so you can snap an infant car seat carrier right onto the carrier frame, enabling you to move baby from car to stroller and back without disrupting sleep.

Brands include: Chicco, Combi, Cosco, Britax, Dorel Juvenile Group (Eddie Bauer), Evenflo, Fisher-Price, Graco, Inglesina, Kolcraft, Maclaren, Pliko, Peg Perego.

LIGHTWEIGHT STROLLERS

Lightweights, aka umbrella strollers, are easy to heft and quick to fold so they're extremely portable. The simple design consists of a simple metal frame with a suspended cloth seat. Two-seater versions are available for twins.

Cost: $40-$99.

Upside: Great for anytime you need to take baby in and out of the car, such as doing errands or traveling. Inexpensive.

Downside: Not appropriate for babies without upper-body control. No suspension, no padding,

Don't skip days; you're more likely to be successful if you develop a routine. Don't think about whether you'll walk today; think about when you'll walk.

and little or no sun protection for baby. Skinny, small wheels roll best on smooth, paved surfaces.

Make sure: You choose a model that weighs under 12 pounds, folds quickly and easily, and stows compactly for easy storage in car or at home.

Nice extras: One-hand folding/setup. A basket underneath to stow gear.

Brands include: Aprica, Chicco, Combi, Graco, Inglesina, Kolcraft, Maclaren.

ALL-TERRAIN STROLLERS

Relatively new to the market, these three- and four-wheelers have the comfort and safety of a standard stroller (padded seats and bars, adjustable seat backs, adjustable hoods) plus features like oversized lugged wheels for traction and a shock-absorption device to soak up bumps and jolts thrown up by uneven terrain. The idea behind them is to bridge the gap between babyhood and toddlerhood, so that parents may end up buying one less stroller. Some can be set up in full recline like a bassinet, for newborns, but then adjust into upright seats (facing either way) even for toddlers.

Models have three or four wheels; on some the front two are closer together, and the front wheel or wheels can be set to swivel or lock. When swiveling they're very turnable, even in tight store aisles. But you'll likely find that even when locked, the front wheel wanders or wobbles at a brisk pace. Models with pneumatic wheels offer more comfort for baby and will be easier to negotiate over curbs and other obstacles.

Cost: $150–$700.

Upside: Built tough to handle high mileage and years of use. Most are designed for newborn through toddler ages.

Downside: Some look sporty but aren't built ruggedly enough to withstand real or repeated off-road use. They may be heavy and cumbersome for in and out of the car, and when you have to lift the front end for tight pivot turns and going up curbs. Also, they're too heavy for running—for that, a three-wheeled jogger stroller (chapter 14) may be the best bet.

Make sure: The model you buy suits your child's age and size now, and for as long as you'd like to use the stroller, and that it's easy to adapt the stroller through each phase of use. If you want to use it for fitness walking, make sure the frame has ample legroom at full stride, is ruggedly built, and comes with a good warranty.

Nice extras: Additional weather protection features, suspension.

Brands include: Britax, Bugaboo, Graco, Kolcraft, Mountain Buggy, Schwinn (by InSTEP), Safety 1st, Zooper.

JOGGING STROLLERS

Not just for runners, these three-wheeled strollers feature lightweight frames, a streamlined design, and big air-filled wheels that make them perfect for walking in all sorts of terrain. See chapter 14, "Gear 505," for a complete rundown.

GOOD QUESTION

How do I pick the best stroller for my family?

It's scary to admit, but there are so many options that it's impossible to say exactly what's best. You should start by thinking about the number of children you have at stroller age (will you want a single, double, or—eeek!—more?). Then consider where you'll use it. If exercise walks (even utilitarian trips, like treks to the grocery store) are going to be a part of the mix, consider one of the "jogger"-type strollers, because they're just so darn easy to push. Here's some advice based on our testing, and that of some our panel of new moms:

1. Test folding, lifting, and loading. Take the stroller through everything you can imagine doing in daily use—fold it, put it in the car trunk, lift it out, unfold it, put in a car seat, load up your toddler, load up the diaper bag. Try it all, and don't overlook bugs in the system. A small inconvenience in the store can turn into a giant headache out on a busy sidewalk with an impatient baby.

2. Always take a test drive. *Always*. Don't assume that a pricey high-end model is going to be great. It may look great. It may have great features, be comfy for baby, be easy to put together and operate, be durable and well crafted—but in the end not be great for brisk walking. It may not track well or have a handlebar that's not comfortable to hold. To be sure, don't just wheel it in a straight line. Put in some weight (a child if you can!) and get up to your real walking speed. Turn sharply and gradually, try different terrain, and in general try to simulate real outdoor use.

3. Seriously consider *fixed* (not swiveling) wheels. Some models have front wheels that swivel but can also be locked in place. The idea is you let them swivel in the grocery store, but lock them straight ahead when cruising down the sidewalk. A good theory, but many of these wheels—even when locked straight—cause the stroller to wobble, chatter, and otherwise not ride straight, a serious bummer for both driver and passenger. During testing this drove us just about batty.

4. Bigger wheels are better. The smaller the wheels, the bumpier the ride and the easier it is to get hung up on small lumps and cracks. With a 12-inch diameter or greater, you'll comfortably clear most obstacles.

5. Air-filled tires give the smoothest ride. If baby comfort and pushing ease are high priorities, go with pneumatic (air-filled) tires. They'll be the least bumpy even on sidewalks.

Our panel of real moms also offered these field-tested recommendations:

- "Next baby, I'm buying one of those lightweight strollers that you can snap the car seat into. With Susie (now two) we had the standard 'system' stroller that's really nice—it took a car seat, which is great for a newborn—but the stroller itself was a pain to get in and out of the car. That was a real issue. And Susie graduated from the car seat/stroller directly to a jogger stroller (much easier to push, with its bigger wheels), so we never really used the 'system' as a stand-alone stroller."

- "We had a really great, not huge, stroller with a flexible restraint system, really big canopy, a number of reclining levels, and it took an infant car seat. I would have deprived myself of my most important walking days if I didn't have a car-seat-friendly stroller. Also, it's not a bad idea to get a cocoon setup for your car seat—great for winter walks!"

- "We bought a car seat and stroller system that neither my husband—nor anyone else who tried—could figure out how to collapse. As a sleep-deprived new mother, the last thing I wanted was to be the only person who could fold up our stroller. The one I would buy next time would obviously collapse easily, and allow me to have the baby facing front or backward—a huge help just in avoiding sun glare, or when you just can't take your eyes off your little one."

Bottom Line: To pick the best stroller for you, first try any "assembly" you'll have to do in normal use—folding and unfolding, strapping in baby, even lifting into your car trunk. Then try it on varied surfaces, at different speeds, making tight turns and cruising straight. Winning features include comfort for baby (of course), but also easy fold-up and storage. Moms planning speedier and longer walks—and their babies—will appreciate lighter weight and larger, air-filled tires, too. As soon as baby is big enough, consider a jogging-style unit.

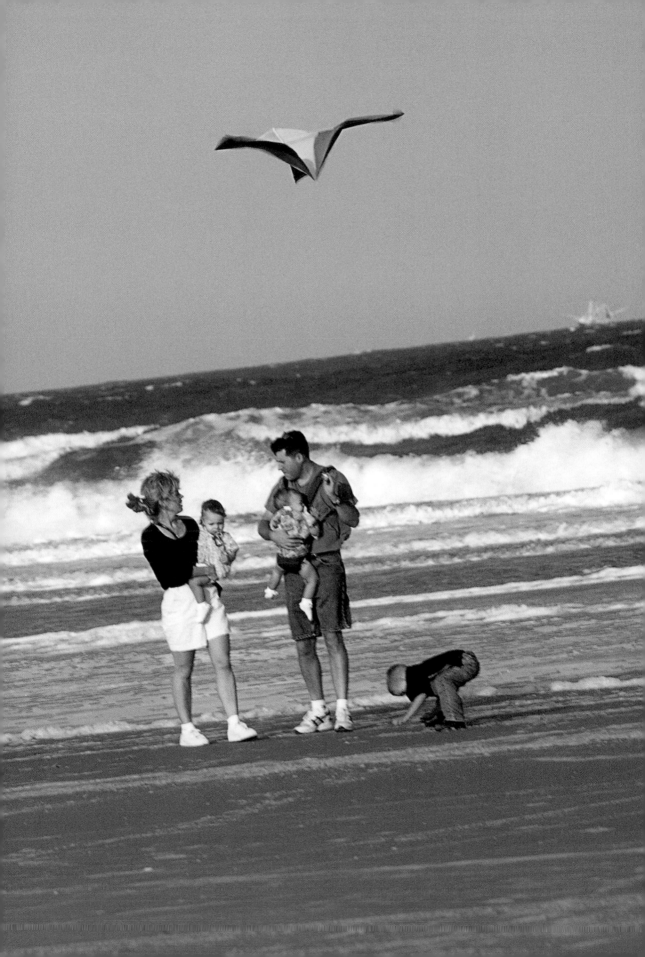

The Walking Program, Postmester I

A Simple Postpartum Reconditioning Routine

About now you may be feeling that your old body is gone, and it's never coming back. But trust that it will happen, as long as you start back to activity very patiently and consistently. Delivery is a serious bit of work, admittedly more for some women than for others, but without a doubt a challenge for all. Depending on how you fared, and any healing required (say, an episiotomy or even C-section), the doctor will dictate exactly how much activity you should do and when. Still, you should share the following postpartum exercises with your practitioner so you can discuss when you can start—sometimes within days of delivery, sometimes after a week or more.

1. **LEG SLIDES.** Begin by lying on your back, with knees comfortably bent and arms at your sides. Place a pillow or cushion beneath your head and shoulders if this is more comfortable. Slowly extend both legs until they're flat on the floor. Then bend your right leg, keeping your right foot flat on the floor and sliding it back toward your buttocks, until your heel is almost beneath your knee. Slowly extend the leg again, then switch sides and repeat. Begin with sets of 5 slides on each leg, building up until you can do 10 on a side; rest, then do 10 more on each side.

2. **HEAD/SHOULDER LIFT.** Begin in the same position as for leg slides. Tighten your abdominal muscles so that the small of your back is on the floor, and raise your head off the floor, hold for a moment, then relax. Do 10 slow repetitions, take a break, then do another set of 10. As you feel stronger (for most women by four to six weeks), you can begin working a bit harder by contracting the muscles more and trying to just get your shoulders off the ground on each lift.

3. **UNWEIGHTED OVERHEAD PRESS.** Begin sitting upright in a chair. Bend your elbows so your hands are up in front of your shoulders. Slowly press your hands straight up (as if lifting an imaginary weight overhead) and then back down. Exhale while pushing up, inhale coming down, keeping your lower back flat. Do 10 presses; relax, then do another set of 10.

The Walking Program, Postmester I

This postmester, you have a few simple goals. Revel in the joy (and, fair enough, the exhaustion) of being a new parent. Slowly reestablish a schedule and rediscover long-lost pleasures you know, indulgences like brushing your teeth, taking a shower, eventually even sleeping through the night. And make sure that daily walking is absolutely, positively a part of that schedule. How fast or far you walk is not remotely important right now. But getting out the door every day possible—very likely with the baby in tow—is about as important as it gets.

How can that be? you ask. *It's going to get so much easier to exercise once this little one is a bit bigger, and sleeping regularly, and then on solid food, and then walking and talking, and able to dress himself, and . . . so on.* To which we say—let's talk about 18 years. Until your bundle of joy is out of the house, you're on an ever-changing but unrelentingly demanding treadmill of parenthood. So rather than wait until it gets easier to exercise, why not just decide that tomorrow is now, and get out for a walk? A slow, sore, stiff, *I-never-thought-I'd-work-as-hard-as-I-did-in-delivery, but-now-I've-made-it* walk. Early in the postmester, 5- and 10-minute strolls are fine. But by the end of three months, you want to actually be reestablishing a very moderate but regular exercise routine, on par with where you were before delivery.

Checklist for Walks with Baby

Don't burden yourself, but do take along enough to assure that you're not going to have to turn around just minutes after stepping outside. Consider the following, along with proper clothes for the season:

- Hat, sunscreen, sunshade for stroller.
- Blanket for warmth.
- "Comforter" for baby. A familiar blankie, say, or stuffed animal.
- Rattle or teething toy, or pacifier if you use one (don't start just for walks).
- Bottle or nursing blanket. Don't be forced to bail just because baby needs a quick snack, but don't leave the bottle in the baby's mouth while riding.
- Minimalist diaper-change setup—optional, but we found it invaluable. You'll need a cloth diaper to serve as a changing surface, clean diaper for baby, and plastic bag with a few wipes (not a full container) able to hold the dirty stuff after the change.

GENERAL REMINDERS FOR POSTMESTER I

- Baby steps first. Depending on your delivery, your doctor will dictate how soon you can start walking again, and how much. But suffice it to say you'll start small and work back *very* gradually.

- Keep it simple. This isn't the time for athletic heroics. You'll probably want to stick with comfortable walks on familiar routes, and speed doesn't matter. Just getting out and moving does.

- Build walking into the day. No two days will be identical, but as the days pass, you'll be getting into more regular sleep and feeding patterns (trust us, it will happen). For some it will take weeks, for others months, but be sure to build walking right back into the schedule as it takes shape. In fact, adding walking will likely help your days shape up sooner!

- Do the brief walking warm up routine (chapter 3) before at least one walk a day.

- Focus on posture, not speed. Distance doesn't matter, but walking with good tall posture does. Don't let using a front carrier or pushing a stroller cause stooped shoulders or an arched lower back.

- Get back to multiple short walks. Though it may seem like a project just to get out the door (*Where's the baby's hat? Where's the front carrier? Where are my shoes? Now where's the baby's hat?*), a few 10-minute walks may be easier on your body. They can also add structure and activity to the day and help give baby healthy doses of daylight and fresh air as you establish sleep and waking times.

- With your doctor's permission, do gentle reconditioning work. The postpartum strength moves will help get muscles toned and back in action.

- Midtrimester, add some stretching. Start with a few of the most comfortable moves. But you'll probably find that if you do the full stretch routine on the floor, with the baby nearby, it can fit into your schedule and is a good addition to the postpartum strength moves.

- Get back to Kegels. Do them as soon as your doctor says so, to firm up your pelvic floor.

LOW-KEY PROGRAM, POSTMESTER I

This is the simple goal: Get onto a life schedule that keeps you and the baby happy, and make walking a part of that schedule.

WEEKLY GOALS FOR THE LOW-KEY PROGRAM

▪ Try to get out for walks five days a week, at least.

▪ Focus on a healthy walking posture and moving at a comfortable pace.

▪ Begin with 5- to 10-minute walks. Add walking minutes very gradually—roughly 10 to 20 percent at a time to your weekly total. So if you did an hour of walking total in one week (six 10-minute walks), boost to an hour and 10 minutes (add 5 minutes to two days) the next.

▪ At this pace, you should easily get back up to fairly regular 20- to 30-minute walks within three months. That's not including the additional time for conditioning and stretching you should be doing.

▪ Break your walks up if this is easier to fit into your life.

▪ Start with the postpartum exercises as soon as the doctor says they're okay, three to five days a week (usually within days of delivery).

▪ If all is well and your doctor says okay, begin adding moves from the full stretch routine from Trimester I (see chapter 3) by weeks six to eight. Add exercises gradually, with the goal of doing the full routine twice a week, by week 13 postpartum.

low-key program

A TYPICAL WEEK NEAR THE END OF POSTMESTER I, LOW-KEY PROGRAM:							
	MON.	TUES.	WED.	THUR.	FRI.	SAT.	SUN.
WALK (minutes)	10, 15	15	20	10, 10	10	30	OFF
OTHER STUFF	POSTPARTUM EXERCISES	FULL FLEX	POSTPARTUM EXERCISES	FULL FLEX	POSTPARTUM EXERCISES	POSTPARTUM EXERCISES	

MODERATE PROGRAM, POSTMESTER I

Begin putting short walks into your days as soon as you can. Then very slowly start building up your walking time. By the end of month three, your goal is to be walking at least 150 minutes a week—the equivalent of five 30-minute walks. Plus, you should be doing an additional 15 to 20 minutes of stretching and the reconditioning moves three days a week or more.

WEEKLY GOALS FOR THE MODERATE PROGRAM

▪ Try to get out for walks five days a week.

▪ Focus on healthy walking posture and moving at a comfortable pace.

▪ Begin with 5- to 10-minute walks; within three months, be back up to regular 25- to 35-minute walks (that's not including time spent stretching or doing reconditioning).

▪ Break your walks up if this is easier to fit into your life.

▪ Start with the postpartum exercises as soon as the doctor says they're okay, four to five days a week (usually within days of delivery).

▪ By six weeks postpartum, start as much of the full stretch routine from Trimester I (see chapter 3) as you and the doctor feel is okay. Add exercises gradually, with the goal of doing the full routine three times a week, by postpartum week 13.

A TYPICAL WEEK NEAR THE END OF POSTMESTER I, MODERATE PROGRAM:							
	MON.	**TUES.**	**WED.**	**THUR.**	**FRI.**	**SAT.**	**SUN.**
WALK (minutes)	25	30	15, 10	25	15	35	OFF
OTHER STUFF	POSTPARTUM EXERCISES	FULL FLEX	POSTPARTUM EXERCISES	FULL FLEX	POSTPARTUM EXERCISES, FULL FLEX	POSTPARTUM EXERCISES	

CHALLENGING PROGRAM, POSTMESTER I

As soon as you're able, begin putting short walks into your days, and very slowly start building up your walking time. By the end of month three, your goal is to be walking 180 minutes a week—averaging almost 30 minutes of walking, six days a week. Plus, you should be doing either the postpartum conditioning moves, the full stretch routine, or both (from 10 to 20 minutes' worth) practically every day to regain your strength and flexibility.

WEEKLY GOALS FOR THE CHALLENGING PROGRAM

- Try to get out for walks six days a week.

- Focus on a healthy walking posture and moving at a comfortable pace.

- Begin with 5- to 10-minute walks; add a little bit every week, so that within three months you're walking six days a week, with several of those strolls lasting 30 to 45 minutes.

- Break your walks up if this is easier to fit into your life.

- Start with the postpartum exercises as soon as the doctor says they're okay, four to five days a week (usually within days of delivery).

- By four to six weeks postpartum, start as much of the full stretch routine from Trimester I (see chapter 3) as you and the doctor feel is okay. Add exercises gradually, with the goal of doing the full routine four times a week, by postpartum week 10.

A TYPICAL WEEK NEAR THE END OF POSTMESTER I, CHALLENGING PROGRAM:							
	MON.	TUES.	WED.	THUR.	FRI.	SAT.	SUN.
WALK (minutes)	25	35	15, 10	30	20	45	OFF
OTHER STUFF	POSTPARTUM EXERCISES, FULL FLEX	POSTPARTUM EXERCISES, FULL FLEX	POSTPARTUM EXERCISES	FULL FLEX	POSTPARTUM EXERCISES, FULL FLEX	POSTPARTUM EXERCISES	

sample exercise diary

WEEK ONE:

Day	Goals	Miles/minutes, when & where?	Stretch? Strength? Other?	How are you feeling? Comments?
Sunday				
Monday				
Tuesday				
Wednesday				
Thursday				
Friday				
Saturday				

WEEK TWO:

Day	Goals	Miles/minutes, when & where?	Stretch? Strength? Other?	How are you feeling? Comments?
Sunday				
Monday				
Tuesday				
Wednesday				
Thursday				
Friday				
Saturday				

WEEK THREE:

Day	Goals	Miles/minutes, when & where?	Stretch? Strength? Other?	How are you feeling? Comments?
Sunday				
Monday				
Tuesday				
Wednesday				
Thursday				
Friday				
Saturday				

WEEK FOUR:

Day	Goals	Miles/minutes, when & where?	Stretch? Strength? Other?	How are you feeling? Comments?
Sunday				
Monday				
Tuesday				
Wednesday				
Thursday				
Friday				
Saturday				

sample exercise diary

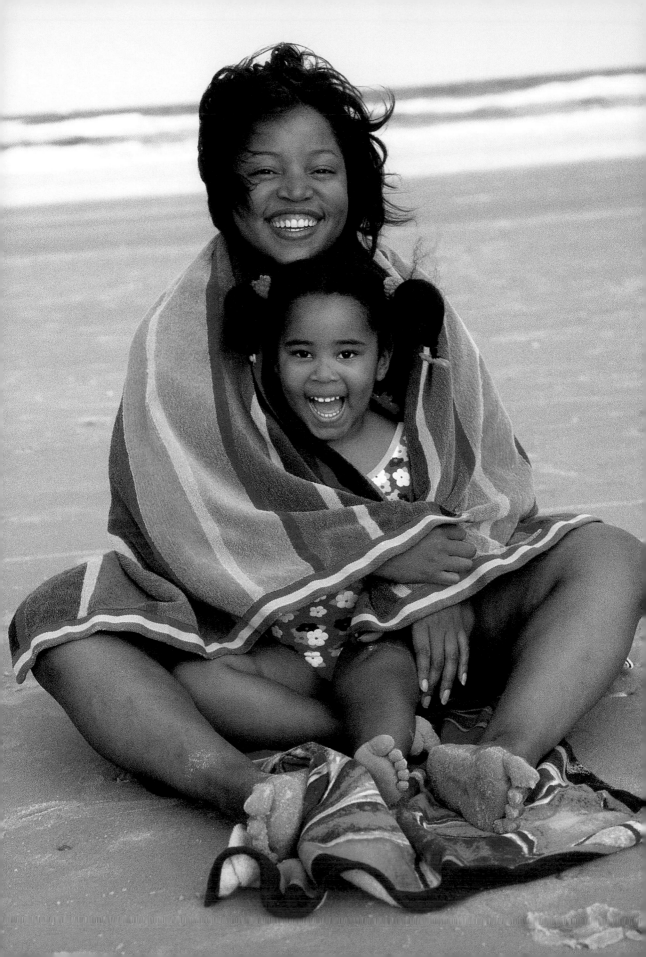

On Your Way to Fitness

Along with Baby May Come the Fittest You Yet

Though pregnancy isn't the time to shoot for a new personal best, you may be surprised to find that after baby has arrived and you've gradually resumed your activity level, workouts actually seem easier than before you got pregnant. Not easier to get to, mind you, but the actual effort required to hit or maintain a certain speed may just seem a bit easier. This phenomenon has been noted by competitive athletes, some of whom even report better performance postpartum. The reason behind this?

When you're pregnant, your heart changes anatomically so that it can handle the larger volume of blood necessary to support the placenta and baby. This doesn't change your ability to handle exercise when you're pregnant, because the baby is utilizing the increased capacity. But "once the baby is born it gets interesting," says Dr. Michelle Mottola. "You're no longer pregnant, but you still have the physiological changes left over from pregnancy." This increased heart stroke volume—literally pumping more blood on each beat—may mean that it's easier for you to adapt to a workout program now, and you might be able to perform better than you did pre-pregnancy.

What if you were sedentary through pregnancy—do you still gain a benefit from this boost in cardiac output? Unfortunately, Dr. Mottola thinks that previously inactive women won't see nearly as much gain: "My gut feeling is that the more active you've been [before delivery], the better adapted your body is." That said, it shouldn't discourage inactive women from starting to exercise now—they still have much to gain. But it's definitely a strong incentive to walk early and often, certainly during pregnancy but especially now that you can reap some of the cardiovascular benefit!

GETTING A HEALTHY PATTERN OF SLEEP

Though your heart may be ready for serious fitness, it may seem your baby has something else in mind entirely. In particular, your household's disrupted sleep patterns may have you feeling like you're destined for anything but a healthy exercise routine. Fortunately, regular walking can be a valuable part of the process of getting you and your child onto a healthy sleep pattern.

Physical activity has been shown by research to increase both the length and depth of your sleep. "Regular physical activity will help both you and the baby get more of the stage-four

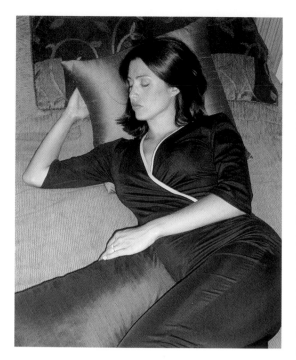

delta sleep," says Ann Halbower, MD, medical director of the Pediatric Sleep Disorders Program at Johns Hopkins University School of Medicine. "That's the deep restorative sleep that helps you recover even from illness or severe fatigue." The result may be that you'll feel a little more reenergized, even on fewer hours of sleep a night, if you're getting daily exercise.

But it's also important to start creating a regular pattern of sleeping and wake, for both you and the baby. One approach is to track the baby's patterns of waking, sleep, feeding, and activity, according to an accepted guru on the subject, Richard Ferber, MD, director of the Center for Pediatric Sleep Disorders at the Children's Hospital in Boston. His book, *Solve Your Child's Sleep Problems*, has been a bible for many parents trying to get some calm into their sleep-deprived lives. He suggests close attention to your child's natural timing of walking, sleep, feeding, and activity throughout the day, and then anticipating the baby's schedule. Be ready to feed when you know baby will be ready to eat. Plan naps for his natural nap windows—often a good time for you to walk. And plan lots of enjoyable stimuli—such as play on the floor—when you know he's going to be primed and awake.

Most important, as the schedule takes shape be consistent. This will only increase its reliability, so that you can count on waking and nap times, you'll help your child have a healthier sleep pattern, and you'll be able to get in your exercise consistently.

How Big Is Baby, Postmester II (4–6 months)?

Your four-month-old probably weighs between 9 and 16 pounds, and may weigh as much as 21 pounds by the six-month mark.

Key milestones: Most babies begin to sleep through the night during this time frame. Head and neck keep getting stronger. Most can lift their head off the mattress to 90 degrees by three months of age, and need less support for the head and neck in a front carrier and while being held. Between four and six months, baby can sit with support, and some can sit independently by six months. Also between four and six months, most are ready to begin eating solid foods. At four months, baby has full color vision, gains some distance vision, and begins batting at and reaching for toys.

What this means for you: The most significant change for many moms is a full night's sleep, leaving you better rested and more energetic during the day, and ready to step up your fitness program. Now that baby has head and neck control, she can ride facing outward (if your front carrier is designed to do this) to check out her surroundings. When baby can sit with support, unveil the jogging stroller. Bring a rattle or toy for baby to hold on the ride.

Great Food for Active, Nursing Moms

What foods make the best milk? It's a question many breast-feeding cultures have invented exotic menus to answer. But the truth is, it's not what you eat, but *who* is eating. As long as you maintain a nutritious diet, only more nursing by your baby will urge your body to make more milk. The following foods won't make more milk, but because your baby's food intake is coming from your body, they'll make your milk, your baby, and you all more healthy.

GOOD BREAST-FEEDING FOOD CHOICES		
WHAT	**WHY**	**WHERE**
IRON	You lost a lot during delivery, which can sap your energy; prevents anemia	Red meat, poultry, seafood
B VITAMINS, IRON, ZINC	Keep energy levels up, carry oxygen in blood	Meats, organ meats, fortified whole grains
OMEGA-3 FATTY ACIDS	Brain builders	Salmon, cod, haddock, tuna
VITAMIN C	Boosts immunity, helps protect body from oxidation damage, increases iron absorption from food	Citrus fruits, tomatoes, kiwi, mangoes, broccoli
CALCIUM	Builds bones, prevents osteoporosis	Milk, broccoli, bone-in sardines, yogurt, cheese
VITAMIN D	Helps body absorb calcium	Fortified milk, sunlight, vitamin supplements
CHOLINE	Enhances memory	Eggs, lean beef
PHYTOCHEMICALS	Promote peak brain function; work as antioxidents	Blueberries, raspberries, blackberries
PROANTHOCYANIDINS (PACs) (BACTERIAL ANTI-ADHESIVES)	Reduce risk of urinary tract infections	Cranberries
PROTEIN	Builds muscles, repairs tissues	Egg whites, milk, grains, beans, meat

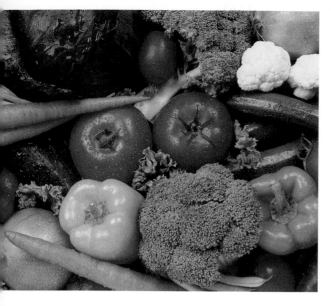

HEALTHY EATING REMINDERS

- Live the clean life. Elements of what you eat and drink end up in your milk, so avoid medicines without doctor's orders, and stay away from recreational drugs and excessive alcohol.

- Get lots of the essentials. Your active body needs them, too, and so much will leave your body through your milk that you need to be extra aware.

- Drink to satisfy your thirst. You may experience more while nursing, but don't drink to feeling bloated. If your urine is concentrated (yellow), up the intake; shoot for the recommended eight glasses of liquid per day as a bare minimum.

- Watch out for caffeine. It's a diuretic, stimulating your kidneys to excrete more fluid, leaving less in the system. (Plus, it might affect baby!) Coffee, tea, and soft drinks are common sources.

- Allow four to six hours for the nutrients in your food to reach your milk.

- Get plenty of sleep. Easier said than done, but fatigue will challenge successful breast-feeding (and exercise will help improve the quality, if not quantity, of your sleep).

- If you're not overweight, add as much as 500 nutritious calories per day to your pre-pregnancy intake.

IS BABY BACKFIRING?

If you're not allergic to what you're eating, it's not likely to cause a problem in baby. But if off and on you sense a change in baby—she's gassy, colicky, spitting up, crying, or refusing to nurse—it could be what you're eating. Here are some common offenders:

Cow's milk.
Eggs.
Citrus fruits.
Wheat
Chocolate.
Cabbage family: broccoli,
    brussels sprouts.
Onions.
Beans.
Herbal teas, tea, coffee, colas.
Garlic.

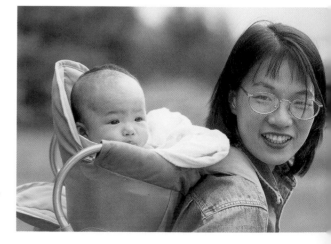

✳TIP:

Walk safe and smart; always walk facing traffic to the left of the road. Always try new walking areas in daylight.

GOOD QUESTION

Is a combination of breast-feeding, exercise, and weight loss safe for my baby and me?

Many women say nursing is not only great for baby, but has the added bonus of helping burn off Mom's extra pregnancy weight. A recent study confirmed that breast-feeding, moderate exercise, and weight loss can mix successfully and safely, as long as a woman is eating a nutritious diet and taking a vitamin B_6 supplement.

The study, at the University of North Carolina, Greensboro, compared two groups of breast-feeding, overweight women (generally 10 to 30 pounds overweight), beginning at four weeks postpartum. One group exercised 45 minutes a day four days a week, and reduced their food intake by 500 calories a day. The other group didn't change habits at all, and both got a vitamin B_6 supplement. Ten weeks later the exercise/diet group had lost roughly 10 pounds, compared to only about 2 pounds for the others. Yet the milk of the exercisers wasn't lacking in nutrients or vitamin B_6, and their babies were growing at the same healthy rate as the nonexercisers' infants. An added bonus—the exercisers saw an impressive 12 percent increase in cardiovascular fitness, compared to just 3 percent (likely due to natural weight loss and baby chasing) for the nonexercisers.

Bottom Line: It's perfectly safe—and quite beneficial—to exercise while you're breast-feeding, as long as you're eating a healthy balanced diet, staying normally hydrated, and trying to get good rest. If you're overweight, it may even be safe to restrict your food intake by as much as 500 calories a day to help with weight loss, but you must talk to your doctor about exactly what's safe for you. And in either case, taking a vitamin B_6 supplement is probably a good idea.

WALKING AND NURSING COMBO GEAR

If you're walking and nursing, don't leave home without this simple setup. All will fit nicely in the undercarriage or back net of a stroller or in a small knapsack.

- A small blanket or cover to toss over your shoulder for a little privacy. Carter's cotton, open-knit receiving blankets offer the coziness of cotton in a very open, breathe-through knit.

- A couple of clean cloth diapers for various wiping-up jobs and to lay baby on when changing.

- At least two spare diapers for the baby (you can jiggle a lot loose on a longer walk).

- A large water bottle, this one not for drinking but for wiping off (with diaper) poopy legs and other assorted appendages so as not to kill too many trees using just . . .

- Wipes. For those last, hygienic wipes.

- Another water bottle, this one for Mom. She may need to be hosed off, too, but that, you will find, can wait; this one's to drink.

- A plastic bag for soiled dipes, et cetera.

- A change of clothes for baby. We found that nursers poop often and in astounding quantities.

- Oh yes, and the baby (he can go *in* the stroller).

TIP:

In a bad mood? Go for a walk! Physical activity can improve mood and energy levels.

Finding Time the Third Time Around

Dana Kilroy, 39, Reno, Nevada

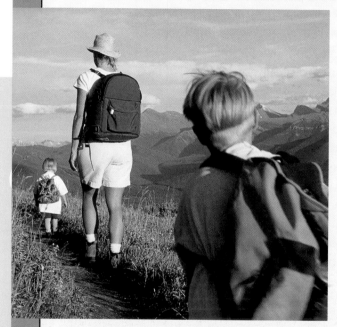

For Dana, staying active takes a bit of creativity. There's not much time left over from caring for Julia, 4, and Liam, 6, and working part time as a freelance writer—plus, when we spoke to her she was dealing with an extra dose of fatigue, being five months pregnant. Unlike her first pregnancy where step classes, prenatal aerobics, and swimming were steady fare, or her second, where she got in a long walk at least five days a week, exercise is now more catch-as-catch-can. She's also hampered by a plate in her leg, courtesy of a 2001 skiing accident that left her on the sidelines for nine months. Still, she's determined to keep moving. "My biggest complaint about pregnancy has always been insomnia, and I find that if I don't get some exercise, the insomnia is definitely worse," she explains.

So Dana squeezes walking in whenever she can. Even if it's only 10 minutes. Even if it's at half her usual pace, because she's got an eye on Liam on his new scooter, Julia in the jogger, and her dog in hand. "Until this year, I never really believed that adage *Something is better than nothing*, but now I certainly do. If a spin around the neighborhood with kids and dog in tow is all I can do, so be it." On a couple of weekdays, she can bank on about 40 minutes, walking Liam to school, which is a mile away, straight uphill. On weekends, weather permitting, the family takes to the nearby mountain desert trails for one- to three-hour jaunts. "It's part of their routine now," says Dana. The kids tote their own water in CamelBak carriers.

Fit to Overcome a C-Section

Being fit was especially beneficial in her first pregnancy. "I was active until the night before I went into labor," she explains, a benefit of choosing an activity as forgiving as walking. Liam arrived via emergency C-section, then spent three weeks in the hospital. "I was at the hospital night and day at first, but once Liam came home,

I started walking again. Being fit made all the difference in the world. In six weeks, I picked up right where I'd left off, doing step aerobics while Liam slept in the car seat, and walking with him in the front pack."

Though everything was different with a baby to care for, walking was an anchor. "It felt like doing something I'd done in my old life," explains

Dana, who was then living in Indianapolis. "I loved that time with him in the Baby Björn or backpack. I'd talk to him, and sing to him, and no matter how cold it was, I'd bundle him up, snuggle him close, and we'd go walk."

Beyond bonding with baby, walking and other workouts provided a critical outlet at a challenging time. "Exercise has always been my number one stress reliever, and juggling motherhood and work was certainly stressful. Exercise became more important than ever."

Exercise Is a Family Affair

"It gets harder to find time to exercise with each successive pregnancy," Dana concludes, "but you can still make it happen." Her advice:

■ Change your mind-set. "If all I have is 30 minutes, I walk for 30 minutes. I don't have the luxury to block out two hours to go to the gym. Some days, it's just a walk with Liam while he rides his bike or scooter. Twice around the block is 10 minutes."

■ Sign up for a class and pay in advance. Dana does a Pilates class once a week. "I go every Wednesday, because it's already paid for."

■ Put in on the calendar. "With our third, I know I'm going to have to make more of a conscious effort to fit it in. I plan to schedule something—whether it's a run or a walk or a bike ride—four times a week, and then squeeze in the rest whenever I can."

■ Replace car trips with walking. "Whenever it's feasible, I allow myself the extra time to walk the 15 minutes up to the coffee shop to meet a friend, and we sometimes walk a mile to the park instead of driving."

■ Have the right gear. With a double and a single jogger, a backpack, snowshoes, a bike, and scooter, Dana's got multiple options for staying active.

4. JOIN A GROUP

There's a reason so many people get together with others to walk—it's a sure path to success. Not only is it more enjoyable, but it's proven to increase the likelihood that you'll exercise regularly. In effect, they act as your walking support group. Walking groups range from formal to casual, and from competitive to social, and most are delighted to have new members. Here are some types you might find in your area (check out "Clubs" on the resource list).

■ **New-mother support groups.** Get more than the scoop on diaper sales, breast-feeding, making your own baby food, and the best sitters; hook up with other moms to walk while you talk.

■ **Worksite walking programs.** If you're heading back to work, make your first stop the fitness center or wellness coordinator and find who else is walking and when. Otherwise, get your own lunchtime walking group started.

■ **Health clubs, fitness centers, YMCAs.** Many have walking classes where you'll get tips on healthy technique and boosting the intensity of your walk; a way to hook up with walking partners.

■ **Parks and recreation departments, community centers, civic and historic groups.** You'll find a broad range of walkers here. Some care most about the walk (exploring local parks and pathways), others more about what you're seeing (historic walks and garden tours, for example).

Hiking and trail organizations. Missions vary—some focus on maintaining a specific trail or educational activities, others on organizing group hikes—but walking is integral to all. Many specifically offer outings for introducing young children to the outdoors. (See "Hiking" on the resource list.)

Racewalking clubs. The high-speed fringe of the walking world, they embrace newcomers and delight in teaching novices. Most gather for weekly workouts at a track and organize occasional races, as much for fun as competition. Some also put together more serious teams for regional and national competitions. A caution: Racewalking will get you in great shape, but it can be addictive. (See "Racewalking" on the resource list.)

Neighborhood groups. Some of the most effective "clubs" are informal groups of neighbors who just like to get together for regular walks. Rustle up some friends and invite them out for a walk; set a specific time and day for a once-a-week outing, or make a phone list so you can call when in need of a partner.

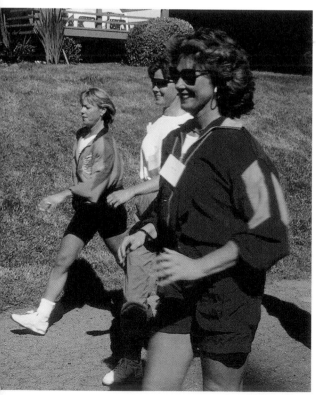

5. ENLIST SUPPORT

Common in successful exercisers, the first step is as simple as this: Tell anyone and everyone you know that you're walking, and ask for their help. Mention it at work, the dinner table, parties, everywhere. The next time someone sees you, they may ask about your walking; you'll walk simply to avoid disappointing them. But even better, you'll enjoy thinking of yourself as an active person—a walker, an athlete. Plus, you'll likely come across new walking partners (a proven exercise booster).

Even if unable to walk with you, others can help you make time for your walks if you're clear that it's a priority. Your spouse can pick up the older kids; coworkers can cut you some slack if you'd rather not do a lunch meeting because that's when you walk; a friend can watch the baby and let you have just 30 minutes to yourself. Most people are happy to help—you just have to ask.

6. MAP OUT OPPORTUNITIES

A simple exercise that the counselors at the Cooper Clinic lead is guaranteed to open your eyes to walking opportunities in your daily life. Get a detailed map of the area around your home (a local real estate map works well) and cut lengths of string equal to 0.5 mile and 1 mile on the map scale. Then draw circles with radii of 0.5 mile (about an 8- to 10-minute walk) and 1 mile (15 to 20 minutes) centered on your home.

Now anytime you're out walking or driving, identify every possible destination that might interest you within these circles, and mark them on the map. Include all of these, and anything else you can think of:

- Bank, ATM.
- Grocery or convenience stores.
- Post office.
- Coffee shop, deli.
- Day care, babysitter's.
- Park, walking trail.
- Playground.
- Bus or transit stop.
- Your friends' homes.
- Your kid's friends' homes.

The final step: Post the map on the fridge as a reminder of all the places you can travel on foot, and try walking to one every day. Too hard? Then

GOOD QUESTION

Are lots of shorter walks really as good for me as one longer one?

It depends on what you mean by good for you. Let's consider the impact in three ways.

Health?

Yes. When it comes to reducing your risk for obesity, heart disease, and other chronic illnesses, several small walks do just as much good as one big one. Consistent daily activity is much more important to your health than how the exercise is spread over the day.

Weight Loss?

Yes! The total number of calories you burn is what matters, not when you burn them (see chapter 16 for calorie burn estimates). Accumulating 60 minutes of walking will burn about 250 to 400 calories, depending on your speed. Whether you do it all at once or in six 10-minute chunks doesn't matter, as long as you go the same speed for the same total time.

Aerobic fitness?

No. How you collect your exercise minutes does matter for aerobic fitness. Shorter exercise bouts aren't likely to get your heart rate up as high, nor to keep it there as long. So they won't offer the same benefits as a continuous brisk walk of 20 minutes or longer.

Bottom Line: Multiple shorter walks are beneficial and can improve your health profile and help with weight loss just as well as one longer walk, as long as the total amount walked is the same. But for improved aerobic fitness, you'll need at least three days a week of continuous brisk walking of more than 20 minutes at a time; lesser walks likely won't challenge your heart enough to build cardiovascular strength. Still, most important is this point: Even a short walk is far better than doing nothing at all.

---

start with one walking destination a week, then every three days, then every day, then two a day, and so on. (If you work outside the home, repeat the exercise near your job, for lunchtime walks.) Eventually you'll have a hard, fit body, know everyone in town by sight, and be ready to sell the car–and buy a new stroller because you've worn yours out.

7. BREAK IT UP

Not everyone finds this a panacea. For some, getting out and walking first thing in the morning is the key to success, and doing it all at once is the only way it will happen. But if you don't have someone else to take care of the baby, or simply don't get chunks of 30 to 60 minutes during your day, breaking up your walks can be a great way to go. It will provide the same health benefits (see the "Good Question" box) and burn about the same number of calories.

This is especially useful after you've tried tip 6, mapping walking destinations near home (and work). Those 10-minute walks for errands throughout the day add up fast.

8. COUNT STEPS—USING A PEDOMETER

Here's this postmester's secret weapon, so get ready: It's time to buy a pedometer. And if you already have one, good news: Now you'll actually know how to use it!

A pedometer is a pager-sized device worn on your waistband that simply records the number of steps you take based on the swing of your hips. Research

TIP:

Back away slowly from threatening dogs. Speak to a scary dog in a calm, firm voice.

GOOD QUESTION

How'd they come up with the goal of walking 10,000 steps per day?

It takes roughly 2,000 steps to walk a mile. In normal daily activity, many people cover about 2 to 3 miles, depending on how active they are. That accounts for about 4,000 to 6,000 steps a day for reasonably active people. To reach 10,000, you'd need to come up with at least another 4,000 steps in a day. That's about 2 miles' worth, or, for somebody walking at a brisk pace—voilà—about a 30-minute walk! So the 10,000-step daily goal is roughly analogous to the surgeon general's recommendation to accumulate at least 30 minutes of activity most days of the week. Plus, "10K a day" trips off the tongue and is an easy target to remember.

But there's a problem with the 10,000-step goal. If you happen to be someone who doesn't take many steps in normal daily life—working at a desk, say, or driving a taxi—then you shouldn't start by shooting for 10,000. If you normally average 3,000 steps a day, then your initial goal might be to try to reach 4,000 or 5,000. When you've mastered that, work up to 7,000 and then eventually 10,000.

Bottom Line: Ten thousand steps is very roughly 5 miles of walking; it's also approximately the amount of daily physical activity that's been shown to reduce risk for chronic disease and an early death in large epidemiological research studies. It's a good eventual goal, but if you've been fairly inactive lately (averaging fewer than 6,000 steps a day), don't jump right up to a 10K-a-day goal. Instead, use the "20 Percent Boost" approach given in this chapter to add steps gradually.

shows that some are surprisingly accurate—counting your real steps, but ignoring your leg jiggling under the table or bumps when riding in the car. They're not especially useful for measuring the distance you walk (unless you calibrate it properly—see chapter 14 for purchase and calibration tips), but they do give a good sense of your total daily activity.

The idea of recording steps all day long began with public health experts in Japan, and it's now all the rage in exercise and weight loss programs across the United States. Most experts recommend that if you can't make time for exercise, at least be sure to get 10,000 steps over the course of each and every day. From a health standpoint, this is the rough equivalent of the surgeon general's recommendation to accumulate 30 minutes of physical activity every day (see the "Good Question" box).

Sneak More Walking into Your Day with a Pedometer

Though 10,000 steps is the recommended amount of daily activity for long-term health, it may not be enough to satisfy your goals. There are three levels of daily activity you can target with a pedometer:

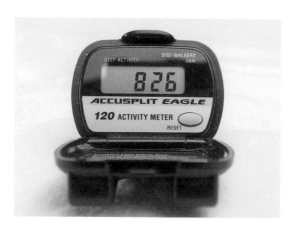

- **Health: 10,000 steps a day.** For a reduced risk of chronic disease and early death, shoot for 10,000 steps per day. Some days can be longer, some shorter, but accumulate 60,000 to 70,000 steps a week and you'll be on your way to health.
- **Weight loss: 12,000–15,000 steps a day.** If you want to peel off the pounds at a more notice-

able rate, boost your daily activity to 12,000 to 15,000 steps, at least a few days of the week. Start at the lower end of the range, but eventually work up to 15,000 whenever you can.

- **Fitness: 3,000 steps fast.** To really strengthen your cardiovascular system, don't just add more steps. Instead, focus on picking up the pace for 2,000 to 4,000 steps, three or more days a week. That means at least 2,000 steps (about a mile) at a speed that gets you breathing hard—so much so that you don't feel like talking, but you're not bent over gasping, either.

A warning, however: Don't try for those step totals right off the bat. The best way to safely increase your daily walking is to first measure how many steps you're taking right now. Then you can gradually add steps every week, until you've worked up to your target. The following five-week program is a great way to safely boost your daily activity totals.

A SIMPLE PEDOMETER WALKING PROGRAM

This program does not focus on measuring the distance you walk. Pedometer distance measures are notoriously inaccurate, especially for all-day wear. That's because the length of your stride varies dramatically. Brisk fitness walking strides taken outside are much longer than shuffling steps around the kitchen or changing table; steps while wearing a front carrier are shorter than without it. (That's why we don't recommend buying a pedometer that estimates distance or—even less accurate—calories burned; just go with a simple, and less expensive, step counter.) If you want distance estimates, see chapter 14; for calorie burn estimates, check out chapter 16.

Begin by wearing your pedometer every day, all day, and using a simple log like the one shown on page 140. Put the pedometer on your hip when you get up in the morning, wear it all day except when submerged in water, and take it off as you climb into bed at night. Every night, record the steps taken that day and write it on the log, then reset the pedometer to zero for the next day.

For the first week—this is very important—don't change your life at all. Just wear the pedometer and keep doing exactly whatever you normally do. If you normally get out for a walk, fine, but don't increase your walking and don't start now if you haven't been walking. Simply live life normally, and record steps for a week. At the end of the week, add up the steps and divide by seven to get your daily average. Multiply that by 1.2, for a 20 percent increase. This is your goal for the next week. So, if at the end of week 1 you averaged 3,000 steps per day, in week 2 you want to shoot for 3,600 daily steps.

The great advantage is that unlike watching the bathroom scale, where it takes forever for the needle to move, you can boost your steps with only a few minutes of effort a day. You can add 100 steps in just a minute of continuous walking; 1,000 steps takes less than 10 minutes. Keep boosting 20 percent a week until you reach the recommended average daily steps for your goal, be it health or weight loss.

☀TIP:

Start an unbroken streak of days on which you've walked for at least 10 minutes.

20% Boost Program for Pedometers

WEEK 1—DON'T CHANGE ANYTHING; JUST MEASURE YOUR TYPICAL DAILY STEPS.

MON.	TUE.	WED.	THUR.	FRI.	SAT.	SUN.	TOTAL STEPS

TOTAL STEPS DIVIDED BY 7 = _____ AVERAGE STEPS
AVERAGE STEPS X 1.2 = _____ GOAL FOR NEXT WEEK

WEEK 2—TRY TO BOOST YOUR DAILY STEPS BY JUST 20%; ADD BITS HERE AND THERE.

MON.	TUE.	WED.	THUR.	FRI.	SAT.	SUN.	TOTAL STEPS

TOTAL STEPS DIVIDED BY 7 = _____ AVERAGE STEPS
AVERAGE STEPS X 1.2 = _____ GOAL FOR NEXT WEEK

WEEK 3—CONTINUE WEEKLY BOOSTS UNTIL YOU REACH 10,000 STEPS A DAY.

MON.	TUE.	WED.	THUR.	FRI.	SAT.	SUN.	TOTAL STEPS

TOTAL STEPS DIVIDED BY 7 = _____ AVERAGE STEPS
AVERAGE STEPS X 1.2 = _____ GOAL FOR NEXT WEEK

WEEK 4—DON'T TRY TO ADD MORE THAN 20% EACH WEEK TO YOUR AVERAGE.

MON.	TUE.	WED.	THUR.	FRI.	SAT.	SUN.	TOTAL STEPS

TOTAL STEPS DIVIDED BY 7 = _____ AVERAGE STEPS
AVERAGE STEPS X 1.2 = _____ GOAL FOR NEXT WEEK

WEEK 5—IF WEIGHT LOSS IS A GOAL, TRY FOR SEVERAL DAYS OF 12,000+ STEPS.

MON.	TUE.	WED.	THUR.	FRI.	SAT.	SUN.	TOTAL STEPS

TOTAL STEPS DIVIDED BY 7 = _____ AVERAGE STEPS
AVERAGE STEPS X 1.2 = _____ GOAL FOR NEXT WEEK

HOW DO I ADD 100 STEPS TO MY DAY?

It only takes a minute, literally! Here are just a
few ideas that will add 100 steps:

- Do jumping jacks, jump rope, or just walk
around the house for the length of a TV commer-
cial break.
- Calm an unsettled baby by walking through
every room in your house (twice, if it's small).
- Go get the mail, take out the trash, bundle up
the recyclables.
- Pace–don't sit–while talking on the telephone.
- Push the stroller down every aisle in the grocery
store, even if you don't have to.

HOW DO I ADD 1,000 STEPS TO MY DAY?

Invest 10 minutes of continuous walking, and
you'll earn more than 1,000 steps. The baby can
join you for almost all of these:

- Walk, rather than drive 10 minutes (or more), to
a friend's house for a play date.
- Vacuum two or three rooms, with vigor (try the
front carrier).
- Intentionally park at the end of the mall farthest
from where you're going.
- Load up the stroller and walk to a corner store
for the newspaper, milk, or bread.
- Take a quick stroll rather than sit down for a
midmorning snack.

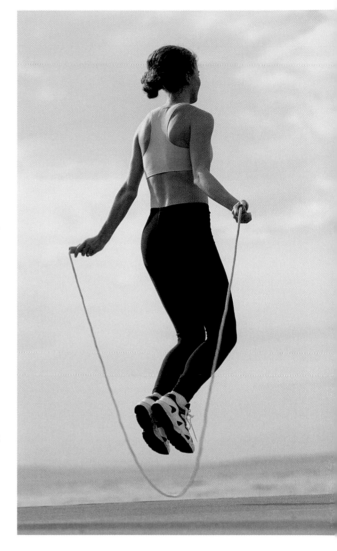

HOW FAST AM I WALKING?

You can actually count how many steps you take in a minute of walking to estimate your speed. (Or count for 20 seconds, and multiply by three.) Or let your
pedometer do the heavy lifting–it will count how many steps you take in exactly
10 minutes of walking. Divide the step total by 10, and you have your average
steps for one minute. Then roughly estimate your speed from the following table
(for more detail, see chapter 16):

STEPS/MINUTE	STEPS IN 20 SECONDS	APPROXIMATE SPEED (mph)	BENEFITS
110–120	40	3 mph	HEALTH
125–135	45	4 mph	WEIGHT LOSS AND HEALTH
145–155	50	4.5+ mph	FITNESS, WEIGHT LOSS, AND HEALTH

World-Class Mom
(and World-Class Athlete)

Joy Fawcett, 35, San Diego, California

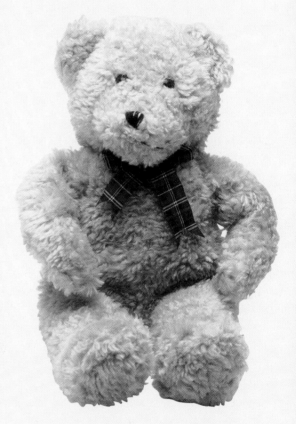

Joy Fawcett has put a new spin on the term *soccer mom*. The first member of the women's national soccer team to continue playing into motherhood, Joy now has three daughters, ages 2, 6, and 9, and is still going full steam. Though two of her teammates are moms now, too, Joy is the only mother of three, and also the only national team member to play the entirety of the '95, '99, and '03 Women's World Cups as well as the '96 and '00 Summer Olympic Games. No doubt she's earned the title of *ultimate soccer mom*.

When she decided to start a family, there was a lot of uncertainty about whether she'd make it back to this level of competition. Would Joy regain her previous fitness and speed? How long would it take? Was it safe to play after having a baby? Could she manage being both mom and player, especially on the road? To stay competitive and keep her spot on the national team, Joy knew she'd have to stay fit throughout her pregnancies. This was especially challenging the first time around.

"I didn't know any other athletes who had done this, and my doctor was conservative," she says. "I played co-ed indoor soccer until I started showing, and then the guys wouldn't let me play because they were too worried." At her doctor's advice, she stopped sprinting at three months, but kept running. With her next two pregnancies, she did a little bit more, so that with the third she was maintaining her regimen of running, sprinting, and weight training.

It was not until her third pregnancy that Joy felt really comfortable that hard exercise wouldn't harm her unborn baby. "With each pregnancy I knew more about what to expect, so I felt like I could push more," she explains. "I read all these horrible things that happened to unborn babies—smoking, drinking, drugs, car accidents—and sometimes even these children were born normal. It made me feel better about exercise," she says. Her biggest concern was overheating. "I made sure I didn't train in the heat of the day, and I monitored my heart rate."

Joy also learned to respect her body's warnings. "I puked for three months with all three, but exercise made me feel better afterward, and I knew I wanted to make it back," she explains.

"Some days you just push through it. Some days you just tell yourself, *Get out and do whatever you can, even if it's a short walk*. I never forced myself to do what my body didn't feel like doing, but I always tried to get some exercise because I wanted to get back to playing."

The Fitness Payoff

Looking back, it's hard for Joy to say whether being fit made labor or delivery easier. "All of my babies came late. After the first two were both 10 days late, I started to wonder whether being fit was such a good idea," she jokes. But once it was time to get back to business, she had no doubt that all the commitment to fitness had paid off. "I started doing sit-ups right away, and usually after the first week I felt good enough to start walking and jogging again." With the firstborn, she was back on the field in three weeks, when a visit to show off her new daughter to her teammates at a nearby practice turned into an impromptu scrimmage. "That might not have been so smart, but I felt fine," she recalls. Bouncing back after baby number three was the easiest. "I think that's because I stayed fitter during that pregnancy," she says. "I felt really good afterward. I was training and running within a week. I couldn't play in a game for six weeks because of concerns about my joints still being lax." But at that point, she resumed playing with the San Diego Spirit.

Just like other moms, Joy has to juggle to fit in workouts. Early on, her own mom helped with child care and she relied on a jogging stroller to squeeze in runs and walks or simply to hold a young baby while she did sprints at a nearby field. Once she was back on the team, the demands of a travel schedule intensified with a baby—and later all three daughters—in tow. "At first I was really conscious of infringing on the other players so I did everything myself. You get used to being extra tired and make adjustments.

My teammates got used to being around babies, and helped carry bags and babysit, and now my kids have a lot of aunts looking out for them," she says appreciatively.

It Isn't Always Easy: Battling Fatigue

Joy recalls two significant times when she started to question whether this was all worth it. Both times, being supertired was a factor. The first time, she and her husband, Walter, had just relocated with their first daughter Katey to Florida, to train with the team prior to the '96 Olympics. "I had four days to get there and find someone to take care of Katey, who had always been cared for by someone in our family," she says. The first morning, she dropped Walter at work, raced to practice, and broke down on the field the moment her coach asked her a question. The second time was this year, when her husband was away traveling and one of her daughters could not be consoled in the middle of the night. "But these moments pass, and I look back and wonder why I got so worked up. Hormones! I always go back, because of all the support I have, and because I love the game." She plans to play through the 2004 Olympics, and then retire.

Looking back, Joy notes that in addition to her obvious love for the game, the support of her teammates and coaches was a huge motivator. "Some people did voice doubts, and they still wonder how I do it, but they've always been supportive," she says. "They called all the time, told me they couldn't wait for me to get back, sent a jogging stroller. It was all very inspiring."

For women who don't have 20 or so teammates cheering them on, Joy offers this advice. "Get fit before you get pregnant so you understand what your body can do and you have a context for when you are pregnant. Talk to your doctor about what you want to do. Trust your body and what it's telling you. And search for inspiration."

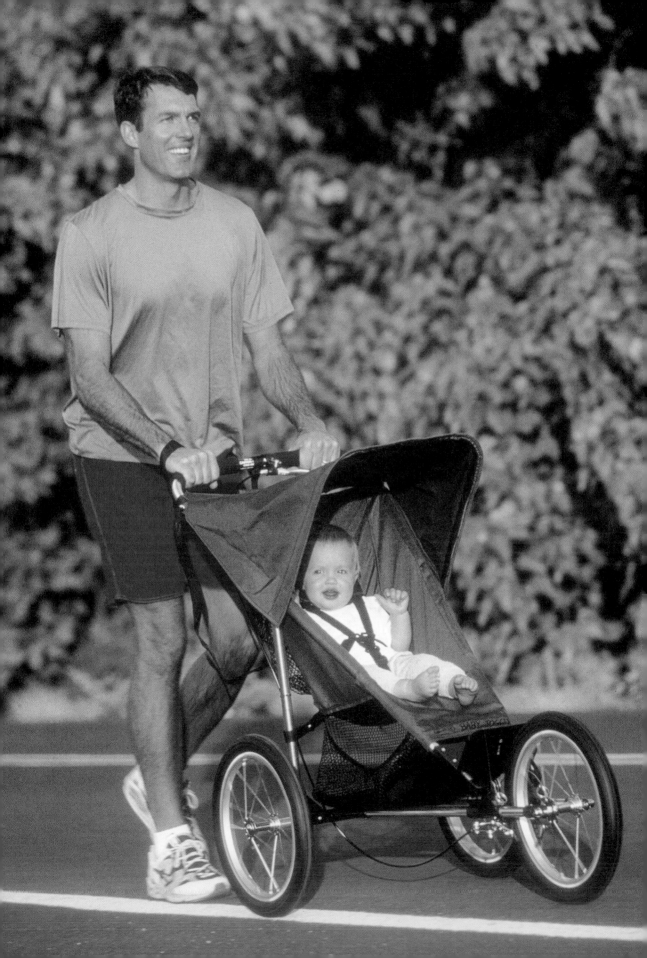

Gear 505: Hit the Road, Jack (and Jill)

Readiness Check: Is Baby Ready to Roll?

By now you may be champing at the bit to get on the road with the sporty jogging stroller that's been parked in the garage for three months or more. First things first. Step number one is to revisit the manufacturer's guidelines for your model and make sure your baby meets them. Next, a development check for baby. Babies don't need to be sitting independently, but they do need head control and upper-body strength before they're ready to ride in a jogger. The timing varies from baby to baby, but most achieve this between five and seven months of age.

You can gauge your baby's strength with the tripod sit: Sit baby on her bottom on the floor, spread her legs a bit, and then put her hands on her knees for support and balance. "Most babies are capable of the tripod sit at five or six months, and then it's okay to use the jogger," says Dr. Rohyans of Ohio State. At this point, it's still important to stick with smooth terrain until baby gains the strength to withstand a bit of jostling and some bumps. "Wait until your child is an independent sitter for trails," adds Rohyans. "That means she should be able to sit independently with no props and grasp a toy that's just within her reach."

JOGGING STROLLER SAFETY

- Follow manufacturer's guidelines for weight and age.
- It's safe when baby has head control and upper-body strength, typically between five and seven months. Gauge with the tripod test (above).
- Stay on smooth terrain until the baby sits independently.
- Always wear the wrist leash, even walking on level ground. Otherwise, if you trip the stroller can get away from you.
- Never wear in-line skates—you may have a blast, but a fall can mean big trouble for your passenger.
- Use the brake to maintain control on downhills.
- Never leave the baby in the stroller unattended.
- When parked (without the baby), set the brake; they roll so easily they can be blown by a light breeze.

Jogging strollers may be odd looking with their tripod stance and jumbo wheels, but they have revolutionized fitness for new parents. Lightweight and agile, these strollers are built for speed. Walkers appreciate these features as much as runners, so even if you never plan to run one step behind your jogger, it's a worthwhile investment.

True jogging strollers are lightweight and streamlined. To achieve this, they are made in a rather minimalist fashion, with fabric seats stitched onto a metal frame of aluminum or steel. Because the seats are generally roomier, less supportive, and offer less flexibility for positioning baby than a traditional stroller, they aren't appropriate for young babies. Babies must have head control and be able to sit with support (typically by six months) to ride in them safely.

Recently, stroller manufacturers have rolled out two variations on the jogger theme. One is three-wheelers that can accommodate babies from birth on up. These sporty strollers (sometimes called all-terrain strollers) have the benefits of support, padding, and comfort for young babies, but may be heavier and less agile than a traditional jogger. And if the wheels are 12 inches or smaller and the stroller has no suspension system, the ride will not be as smooth as that of a true jogger.

The second variation is swivel-wheeled strollers. These sport three wheels (or two in back plus a smaller pair up front), but the front wheel is not fixed. Instead, it swivels and pivots. This does wonders for maneuverability—you can literally turn most of these on a dime, whereas a true jogger requires you to press down on the handlebar to lift the front wheel off the ground and pivot the stroller to change direction. The swivel is great if you're navigating drugstore aisles or turning a zillion corners in an urban setting. But swivel wheelers generally don't track as well as fixed-wheeled versions, even when the front wheel is locked. If you're out to walk for any distance, the resulting wobbly sensation can be downright annoying, and you're better off with a true jogger.

Some jogging strollers include a suspension system that lets parents venture off the pavement with their little passengers. The shock absorbers are similar to the ones you see on mountain bikes, and soak up bumps and dips in the same fashion. If you spend most of your time on smooth pavement, this is an extra you can live without. If you live on a rutted dirt road or love to

Take It from Us:

You'll log lots of miles with a jogging stroller.

"By the time our second child, daughter Skye, arrived, we had a full complement of road gear: umbrella stroller, conventional two-seater, jogger stroller, as well as front carrier and backpack. To put it mildly, we were over the top on baby gear. But with Skye's arrival and Max two and a half years old, I discovered the real and amazing value of the jogger stroller: I could keep up with Max even as he took off on his little two-wheeler with training wheels.

"He'd been wanting a bike for Christmas—'Not a tricycle, Dad, they're for babies'—and so spent the ensuing winter months circling our kitchen/living/dining room circuit, building up his biking legs. (Lisa's duct-taped towel bumpers on all exposed corners and furniture were sights to behold.) By spring he was ready for the 1.5-mile trip downtown, so off we went.

"These trips for errands with the two of them were a panic—dashing along pushing Skye, one hand on the stroller, the other hovering over Max ready to catch a wild veer off the sidewalk. It turned into a killer workout for me, and I'd have never kept up with Max—and kept him safe—if trying to handle a conventional stroller. Plus, he got a great workout, as did Skye who eventually began to insist on getting out and walking once we got downtown. Best of all, by age three and a half (I swear this is true) Max was ready for the training wheels to come off, and now in second grade he insists on riding his bike to school, whatever the weather. Thanks to those early trips with the jogger, we may have created a monster—but a healthy one!

—*Mark*

walk on trails, they make the ride a lot more comfortable for baby.

You might have read that the air filled tires on these strollers inevitably get flats. We might be extremely lucky, but in more than 10 years of combined use of three different joggers in urban and rural settings, along sidewalks, beaches, and trails, we have yet to experience a puncture. The front wheel occasionally works its way out of alignment, but it's easy to fix by unscrewing the bolt on the axle, manually straightening the tire, and retightening the bolt. You will want to keep a bike pump handy to keep the wheels at the proper pressure. **Cost:** $150–$350; more for double and triple models.

Upside: The fixed front wheel tracks straight, allowing you to walk fast without wobbling. Lightweight and minimal materials equal supereasy pushing; great for fast walks and runs. Larger, pneumatic (air-filled) tires provide a cushy ride for your passenger even without an additional suspension system, and can roll over

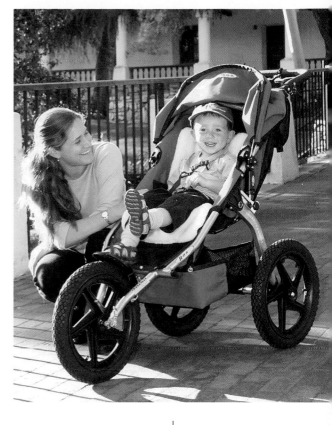

gravel and even sand that would bog down conventional strollers. Most jogging strollers come with long-term (in some cases lifetime) warranties.

Downside: These shouldn't be used until baby gains solid upper-body control. (Some manufacturers offer molded foam inserts and neck supports that help young babies fit into jogging strollers at an earlier age, but it's best to check with your pediatrician before doing this.) The fixed front wheel restricts maneuverability in very tight spaces.

Look for:

- **Safety.** A five-point harness is a must. Also look for two brakes: a foot brake that locks the back wheels in place, and a hand brake with a pin for parking.
- **Seats.** If your child is less than 12 months old, look for reclining seats, which come in handy for keeping younger babies comfortable. Generally, you'll find a seat with an expandable back panel that allows baby to lie back–though not to horizontal.
- **Wheels.** Size matters. For fitness walking and light to moderate running, go with 16-inch wheels. This size is ideal for paved surfaces and gentle trails, and makes curb-hopping a whole lot easier. If your primary surface is dirt, sand, gravel, or uneven terrain, or if you or your partner foresee using the jogger for serious running, opt for 20-inch wheels. Other options include 12 and 24 inches. The 12-inch wheels maneuver well and are fine for zipping about town, but they don't roll as well or absorb as much shock as the larger versions. The 24s aren't necessary unless you're training for the Ironman, or will be on extra-soft sand or rough terrain.

✳TIP:
To improve posture, remember to walk tall, with your gaze forward, not down at the ground. Keep your shoulders relaxed, and gently contract your stomach muscles.

Wheels come in alloy and steel. Alloy resists rusts and is lighter than steel, and you'll probably find that the easier maintenance is well worth the extra money.

▪**Weather protection.** Look for a hood that can unfold to a variety of positions to block the sun, or can be folded back and stowed. The hood should also have a clear panel that gives you a sneak peak at baby below. A clear plastic wind/rain cover (this detaches completely) is sometimes included. Because it lets you go out in virtually all weather, it's worth the money if you have to buy it separately.

Nice extras: Adjustable handlebar height, particularly if you're short and your partner, who also wants to use the jogger, is tall. Suspension, if you plan to go off the pavement regularly.

When you test-drive: Get up to full stride and make sure your feet don't kick the frame. Make sure the handlebar height is comfortable, and if it's not, opt for a model that adjusts.

Brands include: Baby Jogger, B.O.B. Stroller, Dreamer Design, InSTEP, Kelty, Kool Stride, Schwinn (by InSTEP), Kool-Stop.

GOOD QUESTION

How do I calibrate a pedometer to estimate my walking distance?

It's easy to estimate the distance you've walked with a simple step-counting pedometer—and it's probably more accurate than the estimates you get from a more costly pedometer with a distance readout. Here's the simplest approach:

1. Go to a 0.25-mile (four laps to a mile) track, wearing your pedometer, with your standard walking setup—baby in the stroller or front carrier, and so on. This is so you have your most typical stride length.

2. Walk for a few minutes to warm up.

3. Have the pedometer count your steps while you walk four times around the track at your normal walking speed. Or walk one lap, and multiply that step count by four.

4. This figure is your standard "steps per mile." Anytime you take a walk, simply divide the total steps you take by your "steps per mile," and you have an estimate of your total distance walked.

Note: Your stride increases as you walk faster. So if you leave behind the stroller or front carrier, you'll walk faster, and go farther, than this method will estimate. On the other hand, as your child grows and gets heavier, you may slow and shorten your steps, and then this will overestimate your distance. Try recalibrating every two months, to keep up with baby's growth.

A Pedometer Calibration Example

Jan puts her baby in the front carrier, warms up, then wears her pedometer for a walk around the school track; it counts 473 steps. She multiplies by four, to estimate that she takes about 1,892 steps a mile. (For easier math, she calls it 1,900 steps.)

Another day she takes a walk and covers 6,685 steps. Jan divides 6,685 by 1,900 and gets 3.52, or about three and a half miles walked.

If she got a pedometer that needed her step length to estimate distance automatically, she could divide the distance she walked in feet by the number of steps she's taken. A 0.25-mile walk is 1,320 feet long (a mile is 5,280 feet). So Jan divides 1,320 feet by her 473 steps, learning that her steps average 2.79 feet long; she can enter this in the pedometer if she wants it to do the math.

Bottom Line: It's best to focus on changes in your step totals, not on the less reliable distance estimates you get off a pedometer. But a simple approach is to walk a measured mile with the pedometer counting your steps. Then use that step-per-mile figure to calculate the distance you walk anytime based on the step totals.

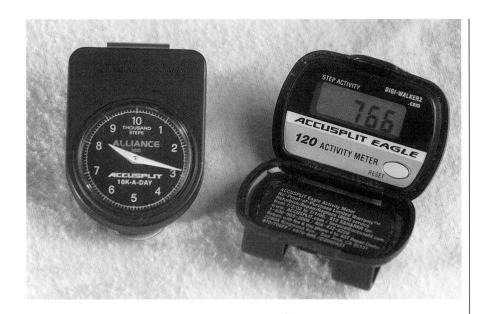

Pedometers

Pedometers range from a simple analog step counter that just shows the number of steps you've taken since the last reset, to an elaborate electronic unit that automatically downloads your step totals to a custom Web site. Fundamentally, they all do the same thing. They're worn on your waist, and a small swing arm inside senses the movement of your hips and counts each step you take. Some are calibrated quite well, to distinguish between bouncing in the car and a true step; others pick up just about any movement. And you can always fake one out simply by holding it in your hand and shaking it.

USER TIPS FOR PEDOMETERS

- Wear a pedometer off center on your waistband, directly in line with one knee; to count bicycling, you can tie it tight to your shoe to pick up pedal strokes.
- Always use a safety cord, to avoid losing your pedometer on the ground or down the toilet (trust us, it happens all the time). Loop a string through the pedometer's belt clip, then pass it through a belt loop or attach it to your clothes with a safety pin.
- Don't get hung up on one day's measurement—instead look for your step trends over time. If on average you're building more steps into your life, then you're doing well.

WHAT KIND OF PEDOMETER TO GET?

There are basically three choices for a pedometer: anolog, digital, and automatic download. Most people are best off right in the middle, with an inexpensive but reliable digital model.

Analog Pedometers

Analogs are the simplest and least expensive pedometers, but also the least accurate. They're especially good if you're buying them for friends and want a cheap way

TIP:

Walking on a soft or uneven surface— sand, broken ground, even water— makes a more challenging workout for your leg muscles and heart.

TIP:

Only wear a
headset in
very familiar
areas. Keep
the volume
low when
walking with
a headset.

to get some other moms involved in your walking campaign; plus, they need no batteries. But they tend to be most easily fooled by incidental movement, and seem to be less accurate on high-waisted or very heavy body types.

Digital Pedometers

The standard for most formal weight loss and exercise programs, the simplest models have an LCD readout showing the current step total, and one reset button to set back to zero at the end of the day. These are reliable, easy to use and read, and can be highly motivating. Added options include:

- Normal watch and stopwatch modes.
- Distance estimates, based on steps; some have two stride settings, for slower- and faster-paced steps.
- Calorie burn estimate based on steps; some also use gender and body weight.
- Pulse monitor, based on finger pulse.

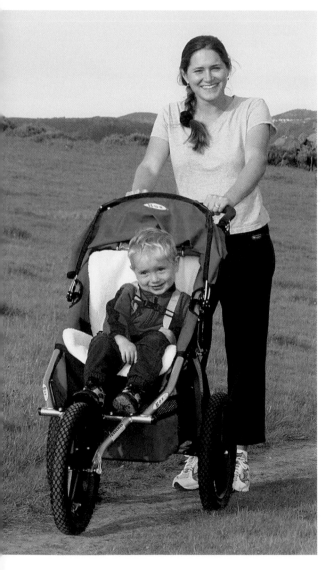

Digital Pedometer with Internet Download

As of this writing, one company, SportBrain, has developed a hip-worn pedometer that you put in a telephone-link cradle at night. It downloads your step totals over phone lines to an Internet Web site with your own personalized page, which allows you to track steps and changes over time, estimate distance and calories burned, and even log on with friends or coworkers to calculate group totals and leaders. It's a great automatic logging system, and lots of analysis functions (averages, trends over times, highs and lows) are available on the Web site.

But it has one huge problem—you can't look at your pedometer and see your step total at that instant; you have to log on to the Web site to see how you're doing. That's fine if you get online regularly, but most time-crunched moms are probably better off with the three Ps: a pedometer, paper, and pencil.

Cost: As little as $10 for simple analog devices; $20–$35 for digital, depending on features you choose; $99 and up for the computer download system.

Brands Include: Accusplit, Freestyle, New-Lifestyles, Optimal Health Products, Oregon Scientific, SportBrain, Sportline.

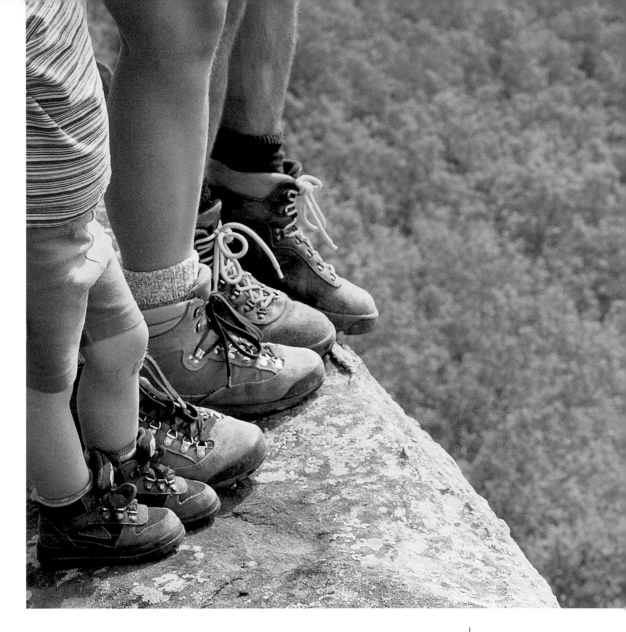

The Future of Performance Measurement?

Some fitness experts believe that the future of personal fitness will be total body measurement systems. Timex has developed a system based on a full-function sport watch that receives data from a chest-strap heart rate monitor and a global positioning satellite (GPS) tracking system worn on your upper arm. The latter actually charts your movement as you walk or run, allowing the watch to display extremely accurate distance and speed information. This Dick Tracyesque innovation is no longer a fantasy, but the deeper question remains—will it really help get more people exercising? Our experience suggests that, like pedometers, if you use it to help build activity into your day—add steps here and there, replace a car trip with walking, boost the intensity in an exercise walk now and then— you'll be successful. Otherwise, this might just be a training aid (and a good one) for hard-core competitive athletes.

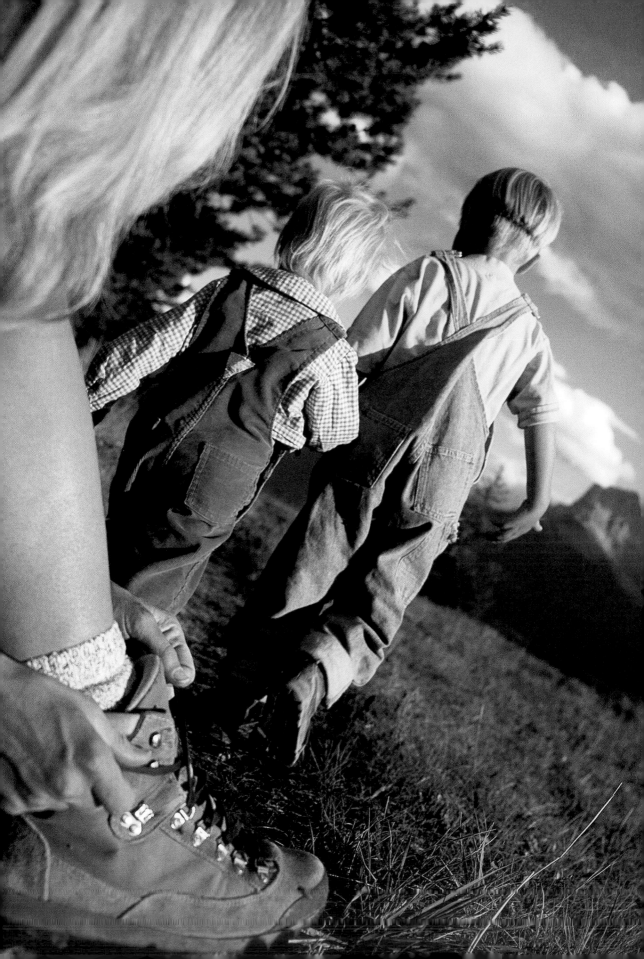

The Walking Program, Postmester II

Climb the Walking Pyramid

Just like the Food Pyramid that's been around all these years, we have a simple "Walking Pyramid" to help you think about whether you're fulfilling all your weekly "activity requirements." As you're establishing patterns with your child, the pyramid can help you think about your goals, and about whether you're doing enough to reach them. It's simple, but based on three very scientifically sound exercise recommendations that are considered standards by the health and fitness community.

THE SURGEON GENERAL'S HEALTH RECOMMENDATION

In 1996, leading researchers surveyed all the existing research literature to come up with the answer to a simple question: *How much do I have to exercise to live a longer, healthier life?* The answer boils down to this: Get 30 minutes of activity most (if not all) days of the week. You can break it up into smaller (say, 10-minute) chunks, but don't miss more than two days a week or you'll be missing some of the benefit. What topped the list of recommended activities? A brisk 1.5- to 2-mile walk.

This is the base of the Walking Pyramid: *Walk daily.* Every American should be at least at this level for long-term health. If you aren't doing anything else, by the end of this postmester you (and your baby?) should be taking at least a 30-minute walk six days of the week, or averaging 10,000 steps per day if you're using a pedometer.

THE INSTITUTE OF MEDICINE'S WEIGHT LOSS/MAINTENANCE GUIDELINES

In 2002, the Institute of Medicine (IOM) tried to answer a thornier question: *How much exercise do I have to do to lose weight?* That's tougher, because what you eat has as much to do with your weight as the amount of calories you burn. Therefore much of the IOM's recommendation focuses on the tenets of a healthy balanced diet, with a strong admonition against zany fad diets.

Its conclusion is that there's a strong correlation between weight loss and exercise. In study after study, the people who are most likely to lose weight and keep it off are the people who improve their diet *and* get consistent daily exercise. In the research, they always outperform the people who lose their weight through diet only. It's because the exercisers maintain their muscle mass—the engines that burn calories all day long—while pure dieters actually lose muscle as they're losing weight, setting themselves up for the inevitable yo-yo bounceback.

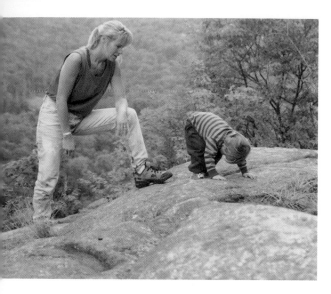

The message is clear—cutting calories can help you lose weight, but exercise is critical to keeping it off. The result is that the IOM recommends one hour of exercise a day, most days of the week. Our experience is that any increase over 30 minutes a day helps boost the calorie burn, and many successful exercisers find that 45 to 60 minutes of brisk walking (not dawdling) at least four or five days a week makes a big difference. So that's what you see at the second level of the pyramid: *Walk longer.* The more you care about losing weight, the more you should try to move to the second level of the pyramid, getting 45- to 60-minute walks (or 12,000 to 15,000 steps) four or more days a week, and 30 minutes (10,000 steps) the remainder.

THE AMERICAN COLLEGE OF SPORTS MEDICINE FITNESS RECOMMENDATIONS

For three decades, this august group of researchers and practitioners has collected the best research on cardiovascular and muscular strength and fitness, and provided training and guidelines to fitness instructors nationwide. The recommendation has three parts, and shows up in three parts of the pyramid:

▪ **AEROBIC FITNESS.** Get 20 to 60 minutes of aerobic activity (such as brisk walking), for three to five days per week, at 60 to 90 percent of your maximum heart rate. Pretty technical to be sure,

but you can boil it down to the two words you see at the top of the pyramid: *Walk faster.* The lower-intensity and longer-duration walks are accounted for by the 30- to 60-minute walks at the bottom and middle levels of pyramid. But if you're looking for top cardio fitness, it's the shorter and faster walks you need. Target a speedy 20 to 30 minutes (or 2,000 to 3,000 steps) two or three days a week to make real progress here. And take heart—these are great calorie burners, too, because of the effort needed to really walk fast. (You'll get plenty more info on picking up the pace in chapter 16.)

▪ **STRENGTH.** The guidelines say you should work the major muscle groups of the body several days per week, doing two sets of each exercise and 8 to 12 repetitions in each set. You can use the program offered in Trimester II (chapter 6), or the one coming up in Postmester III (chapter 18), or another regimen. But this priority is reflected in the second, weight loss level of the pyramid: *Build strength.* Why is it there? Because if you really want to lose weight, you can't afford to lose the muscles that are your big calorie burners. On the contrary, consistent resistance training is as important as longer walks in helping you to burn off the extra pounds and in regaining the tone and body shape you want.

▪ **FLEXIBILITY.** A modest but regular routine of flexibility exercises is recommended not to create much greater flexibility, but to help retain a healthy range of motion and reduce the chance of muscle and joint injury. Because the investment is so small—just a few minutes of static stretching of the major muscle groups—and the payoff so high, this is right at the base of the pyramid and a requirement almost every day: *Stretch often.* It's as simple as the quick stretch routine you learned in chapter 3, but it's got to happen regularly to be of any benefit.

The Walking Pyramid

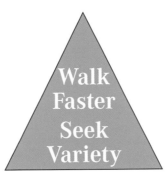

**Walk
Faster
Seek
Variety**

FITNESS   20–30 MINS. FAST 2–3 DAYS/WK. [3,000 STEPS/DAY]

**Walk Longer
Build Strength**

WEIGHT LOSS   45–60 MINUTES 4–5 DAYS/WK. [12,000–15,000 STEPS/DAY]

**Walk Daily
Stretch Often**

HEALTH   30+ MINUTES 6+ DAYS/WK. [10,000 STEPS/DAY]

Begin at the bottom of the pyramid and work your way up, adding more activity as you
feel better and your fitness improves.

Getting Your Walking Body Back

Now that you're carrying or pushing the baby in the stroller and beginning to get back to more vigorous workouts, it's vitally important to keep your spine and torso strong. It's the basis of good posture not just while walking, but in everything you do. Three simple exercises can challenge the front, back, and side muscles that stabilize your spine while offering the least risk of lower-back discomfort—something you're all too familiar with following pregnancy. This is especially important as you carry the baby and he continues to gain weight.

Try adding the 10-minute routine below to your after-walk stretches (or doing them any other time they're convenient) two to four days a week. It will help firm and flatten your tummy as well as help with posture. It also provides a quick and efficient overall strength-building program to complement your walking. Just start gradually—this may be the first hard muscular work you've done since delivery.

THREE-MOVE CORE STRENGTH ROUTINE

1. Curl-ups.

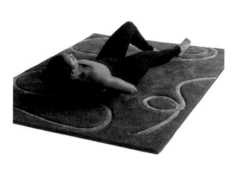

- Lie on your back with one knee bent, the other straight (both feet on the floor), and hands flat beside the small of your back.
- Tighten your stomach so you curl up, lifting your head, shoulders, and upper torso just off the floor. Keep your gaze on a point above you on the ceiling, so your neck stays relaxed.
- Hold the up position for a moment, then relax.
- After 5 repetitions, switch the straight and bent legs, for 10 total.

Ready for more: Start with as few as 10 curl-ups at a time, but work up to 20 or 30 in a row, with all your movements slow and controlled. You can also lift a bit higher for more challenge.

2. Isometric side support.

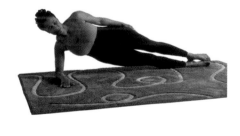

- Lie on your right side, with your body straight, your legs bent back at the knee, your right elbow, hip, and leg on the ground, and your left hip directly above the right.
- Lift your body, supporting yourself only on your right elbow, forearm, and knee. Keep your left arm lying on your straight body.
- Hold for five seconds, breathing slowly and deeply, then rest and switch sides.
- Start with three supports on each side.
- To make these easier, place your left (upper) hand on your right (lower) shoulder to distribute your weight more easily.

Ready for more: Gradually increase to 10 and then 15 seconds in the up position. Then straighten your legs and support yourself like a board all the way from the foot to the elbow (pictured).

3. Alternate extensions.

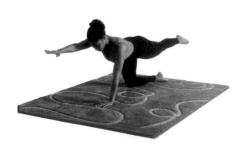

- Start on your hands and knees, and lift your left leg out straight behind you.
- Hold for 5 seconds, then relax and switch legs.
- After three on each side, when lifting your leg also hold the opposite arm out straight in front of you at the same time, for three more repetitions.
- Over time build up to doing up to 10 on each side.

Ready for more: Gradually increase to 10 and then 15 seconds in the up position.

TWO EXERCISES TO PROTECT KNEES AND ANKLES

Burning shins, twisted ankles, and sore knees are three of the most common complaints of walkers of all sorts, from new moms to competitive racewalkers and trail hikers. You're at greatest risk for all of them, and other injuries, when you're trying to boost your walking mileage or speed, or heading onto rougher terrain, and especially when you're carrying a child in a front carrier or backpack. The loosened ligaments of delivery can make you extra vulnerable.

With two simple exercises, you can strengthen and protect these potential problem areas. The first helps prevent a common form of knee pain resulting from your kneecap tracking incorrectly where the bones of the upper and lower leg meet; balancing the strength of the thigh muscles can help prevent this pain. It also toughens your hip flexors, the muscles at the hip that help pull the leg forward and took such a beating near the end of pregnancy. The second move is an all-around ankle and foot strengthener.

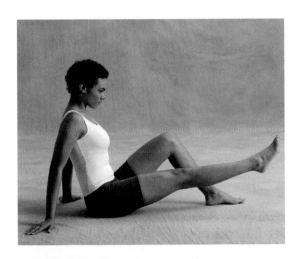

4. Straight-knee leg lifts.

- Sit on the ground with your legs straight in front of you. Bend one knee and place that foot flat on the ground, keeping the other leg straight.
- Contract the thigh muscles of the straight leg so that you see (and feel) your kneecap pull back, making the knee as straight as possible.
- Lift that foot several inches off the ground and hold for a five-count, keeping the knee absolutely straight.

Put the foot down, relax the leg for a second, then repeat the exercise four more times. Then switch legs and repeat. *Ready for more:* As you get more fit, you can gradually work up to 10 repetitions, hold the leg up for longer (up to 10 seconds), and lift the foot up higher (10 to 12 inches).

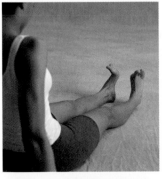
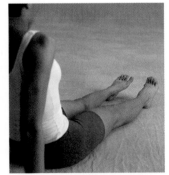
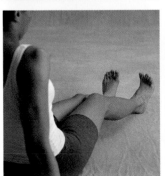
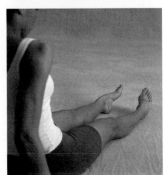

5. Footsies.

These strengthen the foot, ankle, and lower-leg muscles, which get a lot of work on uneven terrain. Sitting on the ground with both legs straight in front of you, forcefully flex the feet into the following four positions, holding each for a five-count, and relaxing momentarily in between. Repeat the cycle 4 times; as you get stronger, work up to 10 cycles.

- First, **up and in**, with toes pulled up toward you, and soles of the feet toward each other.
- Second, **down and out**, with toes away from you, and the soles pushed outward.
- Third, **up and out**, with the toes pulled up, and the soles pushed outward.
- Fourth, **down and in**, with the toes pointed away from you, and the soles pulled inward.

☀ TIP:

Need new shoes? You do if the outsole is worn through, the cushioning has started to compress, your heels lean inward (or outward), or the rubber outsole is peeling away.

The Walking Program, Postmester II

Use the Walking Pyramid to start thinking about your goals. Is your focus long-term health, or do you want more? Is working off some baby weight a priority, or do you want to build top aerobic fitness, too? Your desires should guide how much of the recommended program you do, and which workouts you make a priority. If weight loss is your focus, then don't pass up the longer walks, and be sure to get back to moderate strength training. If you're content with improved health and reduced stress levels, just be sure to get in the daily 30-minute walks.

GENERAL REMINDERS FOR POSTMESTER II

- Stretch every day. We won't even write "quick stretch" in the program notes anymore. Just assume that if we don't recommend the full stretch routine on a given day, then at least you should try to do the quick stretches for a few minutes after your walk.
- Begin boosting your walking time. Now that you've got the routine down and know how to get you and the baby out the door, try adding five minutes to your walks every five to eight days. Unless the baby really doesn't enjoy it, walking time is great time for both of you.
- Add the three core strength and two leg exercises (labeled "core" in the program sample weeks) at least two days a week. These five exercises will take less than 15 minutes; try doing them while playing on the floor with the baby.

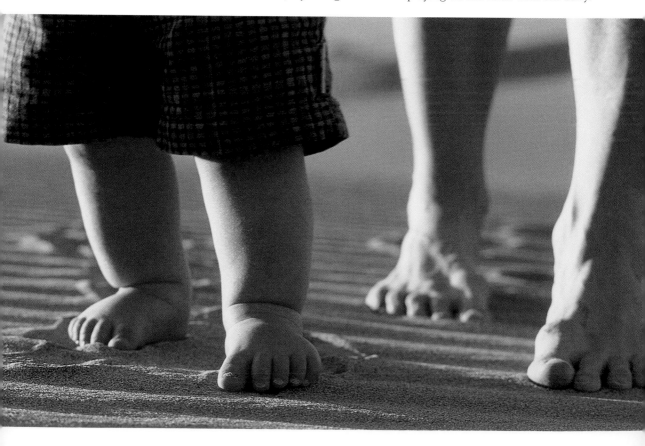

LOW-KEY PROGRAM, POSTMESTER II

Keep adding minutes and making walking a habit for you and your baby.

WEEKLY GOALS BY MONTH SIX POSTPARTUM FOR THE LOW-KEY PROGRAM

▪ Shoot for a total of 160 minutes a week—more than five days of 30 minutes of walking on average.

▪ At least four days a week, shoot for 30 minutes of walking or more, even if it's broken up.

▪ Do the quick stretches after every walk (not shown in the program). At least twice a week, make it the full stretch routine.

▪ Twice a week, try adding the core routine (five exercises). Think of it as playtime on the floor with the baby, or downtime in front of the television, just to keep rebuilding your core strength.

A TYPICAL WEEK NEAR THE END OF POSTMESTER II, LOW-KEY PROGRAM:							
	MON.	TUES.	WED.	THUR.	FRI.	SAT.	SUN.
WALK (minutes)	30	20	15, 15	30	15	35	OFF
OTHER STUFF	CORE		FULL FLEX	CORE		FULL FLEX	

MODERATE PROGRAM, POSTMESTER II

Continue building up your minutes and making walking a habit for you and your baby.

WEEKLY GOALS FOR THE MODERATE PROGRAM

▪ Target a total of about 200 minutes of walking a week—that means you're exceeding the average of six days of walking at least 30 minutes a day.

▪ At least four days a week, shoot for 30 minutes or more of walking, even if it's broken up occasionally. Get in at least one 45-minute walk each week, and do more when you feel up to it.

▪ Do the quick stretches after every walk (not shown in the program). Three days a week, do the full stretch routine.

▪ Three times a week, try adding the core routine (five exercises). Make it playtime on the floor with the baby, or downtime in front of the television. This is important to firming up your stomach and rebuilding your core torso strength.

A TYPICAL WEEK NEAR THE END OF POSTMESTER II, MODERATE PROGRAM:							
	MON.	TUES.	WED.	THUR.	FRI.	SAT.	SUN.
WALK (minutes)	35	30	20, 15	35	20	45	OFF
OTHER STUFF	CORE	FULL FLEX	CORE	FULL FLEX	CORE	FULL FLEX	

CHALLENGING PROGRAM, POSTMESTER II

Don't try to rush your return to pre-pregnancy fitness, but don't be afraid to keep boosting your walking minutes, either. If you're feeling good, you should also return to strength training; at the very least, do the core exercises recommended here, but do more as soon as you feel ready.

WEEKLY GOALS FOR THE CHALLENGING PROGRAM

▪ Target a total of about 210 minutes of walking a week—the equivalent of a 30-minute walk every day of the week.

▪ Shoot for several 30- to 40-minute walks and build up to at least one weekly walk of 55 minutes or more by the end of this postmester.

▪ Do the full stretch routine four days a week (and the quick stretches other days) to rebuild your strength and flexibility; this is an important injury-prevention activity as you continue to build your walking mileage.

▪ Four days a week, do the core routine (five exercises). Make it playtime on the floor with the baby, or downtime in front of the television. This will firm your stomach and rebuild your core strength, and get you ready for more strength work as soon as you feel you can handle it.

A TYPICAL WEEK NEAR THE END OF POSTMESTER II, CHALLENGING PROGRAM:

	MON.	TUES.	WED.	THUR.	FRI.	SAT.	SUN.
WALK (minutes)	35	25	40	30	25	55	OFF
OTHER STUFF	CORE, FULL FLEX	FULL FLEX	CORE	FULL FLEX	CORE, FULL FLEX	CORE	

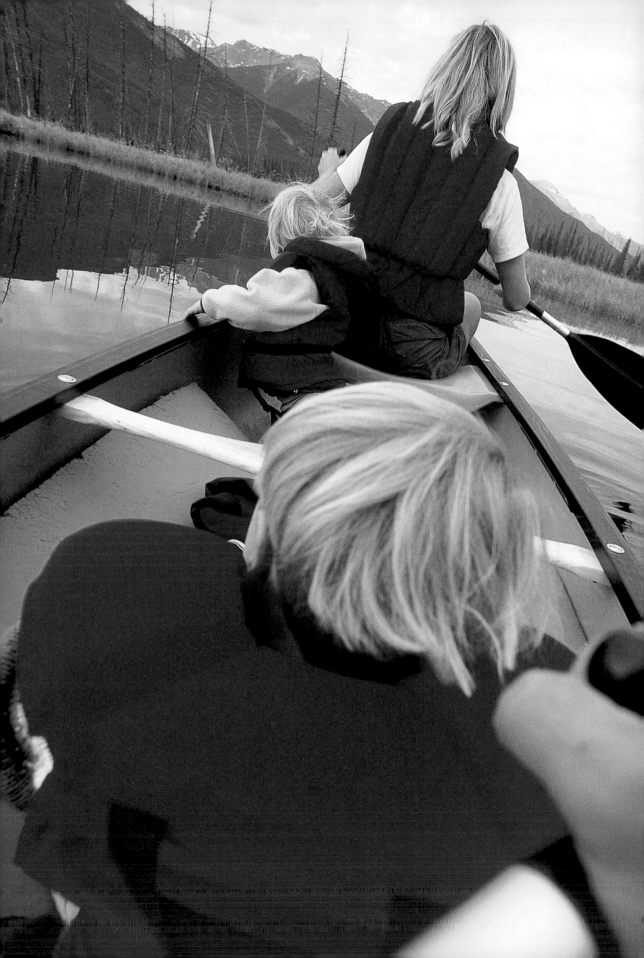

Becoming Active for Life

It's Not Just About Exercise

Now is the time you're going to get some real philosophy from us. All along we've been pretending this is just another fitness book. It preys on pragmatic fears and concerns. *Will I gain too much weight during pregnancy, or not be able to get it off after the baby arrives? Will I be strong enough for delivery, and am I as healthy and strong as I need to be for my baby?* So it's been packaged up with training times, warm-ups and stretches, strength routines; all the standard exercise stuff. Unfortunately, that won't be enough to keep you and your child healthy for a lifetime. It's a good start, but you'll need more. That's where our philosophy comes in.

First, it's our sincere belief that you should wake up every day not wondering *whether* you'll walk that day, but *when*. Know that you're going to walk every day because of how easy it is to do, and how good it makes you (and your child) feel. But not every day is the same, and it won't always be easy. So you need a varied approach to make sure a walk happens every day.

Second, some people believe walking can't be a "serious" workout. Sure, it's been fine for when you're pregnant or have just had a baby, because you can't really do anything else anyway. But it's not intense enough to really get you back into shape. For that, you'll have to run or do aerobics; you know, a *real* workout. Well, they're wrong, and we'll make sure you can turn a walk into a workout anytime you want.

All your walks should essentially fall into one of four categories. Make sure you have a mix of these walks in every week and you'll be on your way to a lifetime of fitness. Depend on only one type, however, and you may find you soon get stuck in a rut.

1. UTILITARIAN WALKS

The most underrated, but perhaps the best way to wedge activity into your busiest days. Put the baby in the jogger stroller or the backpack and cruise to the store, bank, and post office; arrive at home with groceries for dinner and a great walk under your belt. It's not quite as fast as driving in the car, but far more beneficial to you, your baby, and the environment. (You know, the environment your child's going to inherit in a couple of decades?) Many women will have to drive somewhere and park to do this, but that's a good way to choose where you'll do errands—if you can walk there, hitting multiple targets from one parking space, then you're willing to shop there!

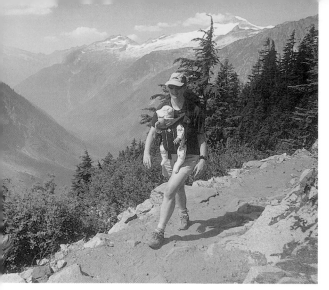

2. LONG WALKS AND HIKES

These longer (45 minutes or more) walks are such a joy they're well worth the effort to squeeze into your week one way or another. Not only relaxing, if you hold a moderate pace (3.5 mph or faster) they can be super calorie burners, too. A long walk is all the more effective if you put some rolling terrain into the mix; a trail over hills can boost the calorie burn by anywhere from 15 to well over 50 percent, even if you slow down a bit due to the climb (see the table). Plus, your legs muscles get added strength work. For more on gear for hiking with baby, see chapter 17.

INCREASE IN CALORIE BURN WALKING UPHILL, COMPARED TO WALKING ON LEVEL GROUND				
	% INCLINE			
	6% (SLIGHT)	10% (NOTICEABLE)	15% (MODERATE)	20% (STEEP)
WALKING SPEED	3.5 MPH	3.0 MPH	2.5 MPH	2.0 MPH
INCREASE IN ENERGY EXPANDED	16%	52%	67%	70%

3. SHORT SUPERFAST WALKS

Don't suffer from the "if it's not 30 minutes, then it's not worth walking" syndrome. If you can get out the door and crank around the block for 20 minutes—even 15 or 10—then it's vastly better than doing nothing. Go fast enough, and it will be one of your best workouts of the week. Not sure you can walk fast enough to even get breathing hard in 15 minutes? Just a few technique tips (later in this chapter) will have you flying through a walk—without nearly the injury risk of running.

4. LEISURELY STROLLS

Not fast, not long, and not even going somewhere useful—once in a while, it's nice to walk just to be out there. This kind of walk will become especially important over the next six months or so as your child asks to get out of the stroller and walk along with you once in a while. You don't want be counting calories then—just watching how fast your little one is growing up.

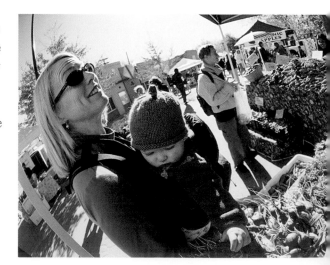

More Workout in Less Time: Walking Fast

When you only have 15 to 30 minutes for a walk, you can still make it a serious workout. The key is to really pick up the pace. Walking fast may seem easier if you don't have a baby in tow, but if the goal is to boost your heart rate and get a better workout, pushing a stroller or carrying the baby backpack is a great way to get a leg-burning, lung-searing effort. With baby or without, here are four technique tips for healthy and speedy walking.

1. WALK AS TALL AS YOU CAN

Keep an upright, comfortable posture and you'll keep your rib cage open for more easy breathing, and your lower back and hips will be set for a quick, powerful stride. A slouch or roll in your shoulders, a forward lean from the hips, or an arch in your lower back can all undermine your walking power.

Tips

- Keep your head level, and gaze forward. Drop only your eyes to check your footing; don't lower your chin.
- Relax your neck, back, and shoulders.
- Keep your stomach muscles gently contracted and your lower back fairly flat.
- When pushing a stroller, be careful not to lean into the handle too much; stay tall.

2. FASTER STEPS

The most important variable for fast walking is faster steps. On your fastest walks, consider counting steps occasionally, with a goal of walking at least 135 steps a minute (roughly 4.0 mph). When you've mastered that, set 150 steps per minute as your next goal (better than 4.5 mph!).

Tips

- Take a comfortable stride so your feet touch down practically beneath you, not way out in front. Don't reach for a longer stride; let it come naturally.
- Focus on smooth, quick steps, and think about pulling your leg forward as quickly as you can as soon as your foot leaves the ground.

 TIP:

Extending your walk from 30 minutes to 40 minutes would increase your calorie burn by 33%, plus add to the after-exercise burn.

How Big Is Baby, Postmester III (7–9 months)?

At seven months, most babies weigh from 12 to 21 pounds, and at nine months, from 15 to 24 pounds.

Key milestones: Sits independently, generally by six to seven months. May begin crawling between six and nine months. Gradually expands repertoire of foods, and may start finger foods around seven months. Distance vision is significantly improved by seven months.

What this means for you: When baby sits well, break out the backpack for more terrain options. At this point, you can also take the jogger on rougher surfaces, such as gravel or dirt roads, paths, and trails. For outings of more than 30 minutes, bring a healthy snack for older babies, just in case.

Having Kids Could Make You a Better Exerciser!

Kim Sutton, 39, Lexington, Massachusetts

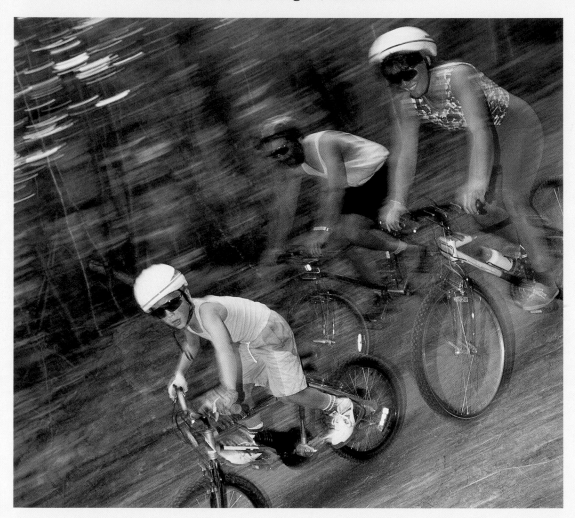

A former runner and mother of three kids ages 3 to 8, Kim faithfully walked through nearly all three pregnancies. "Having kids actually improved my exercise plan," she says. "When I switched to walking, I ended up exercising longer, and because I wasn't working then, I had the whole day to fit in what I had intended to do all along."

Her first son wasn't the world's best napper. "He needed motion," says Kim. "First I drove in the car, then I tried walking." That was the genesis of a habit that spanned six years. For almost every afternoon nap, through two more pregnancies, Kim walked from an hour to an hour and 45 minutes.

"I simply started to walk my running route, and it took longer to walk it," she explains. For her second and third pregnancies, nap time coincided with school time for the older one (and then two), so she always had the window to go. "I had a rain/wind hood and a great fleece blanket for the jogger," she explains. "I found ways to get out most days, and only had to turn back if a thunderstorm popped up."

Nap time may not be ideal for everyone. For some moms, it's hard to pass up the chance to fold laundry, squeeze in some work, or make phone calls. "For me, it just became such a habit. If I didn't do it, I felt more stressed than I would have if I had caught up in the house. I can fold laundry at night, but I can't go for a walk then."

Kim cut back on the length of her walks toward the birth of her second son. "I remember holding my arms out to the side because of the throbbing and swelling fingers," she says. She intended to walk through her entire third pregnancy, too, but placenta previa restricted all her activity after the seventh month. "Suddenly, there was no outlet. I wanted to crawl out of my skin!"

This period of inactivity gave her a clear point to see that fitness was key to a smooth recovery. Despite the fact that she had a C-section this time, she feels strongly that consistent walking for the first two deliveries made a big difference. "Even carrying her and going up and down the stairs was tough, and it was slow going at first when I started walking again," Kim says. But as soon as her doctor gave her clearance, she was off again, and soon resumed her regular long walks. "I had the mind-set that I was going to do the same hour-plus walks again, as soon as I got the okay."

Now that she's resumed working full time, it's much more challenging to find the time to walk, with she and the three kids out of the house by 7:45 AM and home around 6 PM. "I try to get up early and go. It's hard on the heels of too little sleep, especially when the days are short and it's dark so late. But my husband and I just bought a treadmill. Now if I miss that morning window, I have another option." On weekends, walking is a priority on both days. "Mark is great about this. He bends over backward to help me fit it in," she says.

Her children also understand that exercise is important. "They are definitely learning by the example. I don't talk about weight control, but I tell them that it helps me stay healthy and it's fun for me," explains Kim. The Suttons reinforce this message by doing group outings—walks, bike rides, cross-country skiing—when they can. "It's tough right now because our daughter is at that tricky place where she's too big to ride, but too small to go far, so sometimes we split up into smaller groups," says Kim. "But we keep trying."

Kim's Strategies for Making a Walk Happen

■ Nap time is walk time for Kim. It's a reliable slot most days.

■ Look into a treadmill to add flexibility.

■ Work together with your spouse to find time when you get exercise alone.

■ Plan active outings with your family on weekends.

■ Recognize how important walking can be for stress relief. That alone might motivate you to make it happen.

■ Move to a town center. It may sound extreme, but it serves up plenty of opportunity for small chunks of walking. The Suttons moved to the center of a large town when their youngest had just turned one. "One of the main reasons we moved here was to spend less time in the car and to get more exercise. I started doing errands on foot, and we take the kids on foot to the library, park, and town pool."

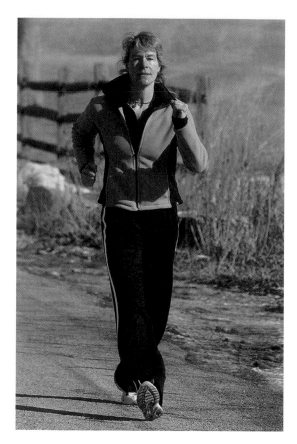

3. BEND YOUR ARMS

The best way to have quick steps is to have a quick, powerful, and compact arm swing. The arms and legs always move together, and faster arms will make faster legs.

If you're pushing a stroller, this may not seem to matter—but walking with a speedy jogging stroller, you'll find you only need one hand on the handle at a time (that's how runners do it). So bend your arms 90 degrees, making them shorter pendulums, which swing faster than long ones. For proof, think of the weight that hangs below a grandfather clock. The height is adjustable to control the accuracy of the clock. The clock repairman's rule is simple: "Lower is slower." Lower the weight, make the pendulum longer, and it swings more slowly—exactly what you *don't* want to happen when walking fast. So bend your arms to shorten the pendulum and swing your arms faster. It's why you never see someone out running with straight arms—it's not just goofy looking, but inefficient, too.

Tips

- Bend your arms 90 degrees (a right angle) at the elbow.
- Keep the elbow fixed (imagine it's in a cast); don't let your elbow swing open and closed as the arm swings.
- Have your hands trace a compact arc from waistband height on the back swing to chest height in the front.
- Bring your hands to the centerline of your body, but not across it in front.

4. PUSH OFF FOR POWER

Generating a lot of push at the end of each step helps in two ways—you produce more forward drive with each stride, and you help your leg swing forward quickly for the next step. The very tip of your toe should be the last thing to leave the ground on each step. Here's a sign you're doing it right: You should be able to see wear on the bottom of your sneaker all the way up to your big toe. If not, you're not pushing off enough.

Tips

- Feel your foot roll smoothly from the heel all the way through the toes.
- Consciously push off with your toes at the end of every step.
- Feel like you're showing someone behind you the sole of your shoe at the end of each stride.

How Fast Are You Walking?

These techniques will boost your speed anytime you're walking—not just during hard workouts. All (or some, if you're a wee bit self-conscious about bending your arms) will work for a quick stroll to the corner store or just walking in from the parking lot to the office. To see if they're working, count your steps to estimate your walking speed. Count every step for a minute, or count for 20 seconds and multiply by three (see page 62). (If you're really flying, count only left or right footsteps, and double the answer.) If you hit 3.0 to 3.5 mph, you're in the health-inducing range; 3.5 to 4.0 mph adds a boost to weight loss; and above 4.0 mph, you'll really start rebuilding your aerobic fitness.

TIP:

Add intervals to your walk: Try breaking up your walk with several short bursts of speed—say, between two phone poles. You'll burn more calories and improve your cardio-vascular fitness.

Take It from Us:

Your energy will return. We promise.

Exercise got a whole lot easier for me once my babies were weaned. Nursing twins was physically and logistically demanding in and of itself. With a chest larger than I ever thought humanly possible, it was just plain uncomfortable to exercise with much intensity, no matter what bra I tried. More importantly, I was worn out from producing so much milk, and it seemed I needed to stuff something in my mouth every 30 minutes just to keep up. Plus, the elaborate system of props and supports and seats that I needed to nurse twins didn't exactly lend itself to say, a midwalk feeding on a park bench. With mixed feelings, we switched to bottles and formula at about six months. Probably not coincidentally, this was the point when I found the energy and comfort to ramp up my fitness program, taking longer and speedier walks, and add weight training.

"Now, I don't recommend cutting breast-feeding short, and the experts all agree that going to a year is optimal for both your health and the baby's. But you can be confident that you're not a weenie, nor are your athletic talents permanently impaired, just because you've had a baby and you're not feeling your full pre-pregnancy athletic prowess. Especially if you're breast-feeding, your body's just working really hard all the time. Rest assured that you will come back as strong as ever, if not stronger.

—Tracy

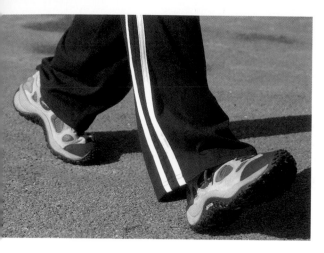

FIGURE OUT YOUR CALORIE BURN

The number of calories you burn during exercise depends on a lot of things—how hard you're working, your fitness level, your weight and how much you're carrying or pushing in a stroller, even conditions like wind or hills. So standard estimates of the calories you burn during exercise can vary from okay to pretty crummy, depending on what's taken into account. The calorie read-outs on most machines at the gym aren't worth the price of their little blinking LEDs. On the other hand, estimates that consider your weight and heart rate (some heart rate monitors do this, for example) can be fairly good.

Use your walking speed (based on a step rate estimate or by walking on a measured course) and the table below to estimate the calories you burn while walking for 30 minutes. Use the weight column that's closest to yours, or estimate between the two closest values. These estimates are on level ground, without any load; pushing a stroller could increase the energy expended by 10 percent or more; carrying a baby backpack, especially on hills, could boost it by much more. These won't be perfect estimates, but they will help you compare yourself from one walk to the next.

ESTIMATED CALORIE BURN FOR 30 MINUTES OF WALKING							
SPEED (MPH)	TIME TO WALK 1 MILE (MIN:SEC)	BODY WEIGHT					
		100 LBS.	125 LBS.	150 LBS.	175 LBS.	200 LBS.	250 LBS.
2.0	30:00	63	80	95	110	126	158
2.5	24:00	74	92	110	128	147	183
3.0	20:00	86	108	129	151	172	215
3.5	17:10	103	128	154	180	205	257
4.0	15:00	125	156	187	218	250	311
4.5	13:20	154	193	231	270	308	385
5.0	12:00	196	245	293	342	391	490

DON'T MAKE THESE MISTAKES

Picking up the pace and making your walk more athletic is great for your heart and lungs, but it can be tough on your legs, hips, back, and shoulders if you let your walking technique get sloppy. And given all your body's been through lately, it's possible you've got some postural habits that are worth straightening up. So give your technique the once-over. Whether you watch yourself in a storefront window or hop on a treadmill in front of a mirror, watch out for these five common errors, and apply the corrections as needed.

Error 1. Looking for Spare Change: Head down, shoulders slouched.

Warning signs: Tightness and fatigue in the upper back, neck, and shoulders; often caused by pushing a stroller or wearing a front carrier.

How to fix it?

▪ Get your eyes on the horizon. If your gaze is off in the distance, not down at your own feet or the ground just in front of you, it will tend to pull your whole body more upright.

▪ Pull your shoulders back and chest forward.

▪ Make sure front carrier is adjusted properly, and baby is riding comfortably.

Error 2. Goose-Stepping: Taking an extra-long stride.

Warning signs: Sore shins, tightness in the hamstrings (back of the thigh), and a jarring thud on every step.

How to fix it?

▪ Think rolling, not bouncing, from one step to the next. Try to put your foot down as fast as you can.

▪ Don't reach for the longest possible stride, and don't let your heels slam into the ground on each step.

▪ Feel like you're gliding along the ground. If someone saw only your head over a hedge, it should look more like you're riding a bike, not running.

Error 3. Chicken-Wings: Elbows flailing out to the sides as you bend your arms.

Warning signs: You can't walk near a wall or a partner without banging an elbow.

How to fix it?

▪ Feel your thumb rub the waistband of your pants as your hand swings back, then stop it there. (Don't let it swing back any farther.)

▪ Imagine you're trying to elbow someone directly behind you.

▪ Don't let your hips have an exaggerated side-to-side sashay.

▪ Walk very near to a wall or hedge—the closer the better. Negative reinforcement will tuck those elbows in.

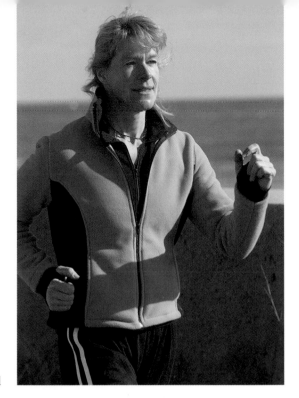

Error 4. Shelf-Butt: Excessive arch in the lower back, causing your rear end to lag behind (often a leftover from the arched lower back of pregnancy days).

Warning signs: Tightness in the lower back and upper gluteal muscles.

How to fix it?

▪ Get your abdominal muscles back in shape, to flatten your lower back. Do the core strength routine more often.

▪ Keep your rear end tucked underneath you; consciously pull it under by gently tightening your stomach muscles and flattening your belly.

Error 5. Boxing: Driving the arms high— to shoulder height or above—in front.

Warning signs: Tired shoulders; seeing your hands swing up into view on every step.

How to fix it?

▪ Think about a quick, compact arm swing.

▪ In front, your hands should only come up to chest height—if you're looking forward, that's just into your peripheral vision but no higher.

▪ Fix your elbow bend at 90 degrees; don't open and close the angle of your elbow.

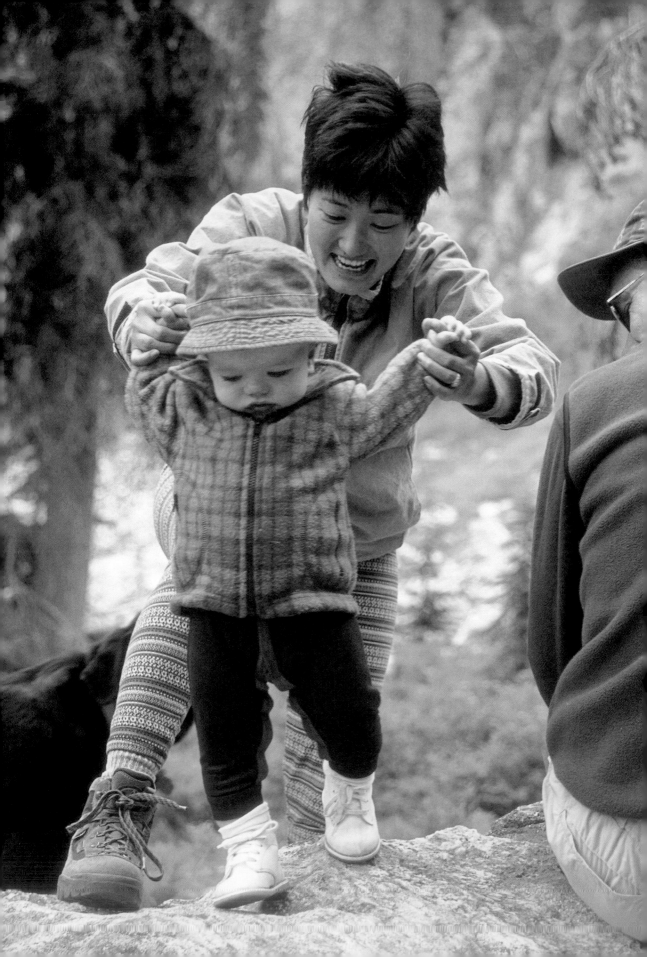

17

Gear 606: Gearing Up for the Trail

Baby Backpacks

There are places that even the most rugged stroller just can't go. And there are times when you need to have baby safely with you, yet have complete use of your hands. For said places and times, you'll find it essential to have a backpack-style carrier. These carriers have a metal frame with a slinglike seat for baby and a backpack-style strap system that holds the carrier on your back. They're designed for older babies and toddlers who have the upper-body control and balance to stay safe and comfortable in a pack's cockpit. Though backpack carriers have been known to make some pretty incredible trips—trekking in Nepal, hiking in the Rockies—they're equally handy for day hikes and trips to the supermarket or park.

The best carriers show thought for the safety and comfort of both child (awake and asleep) and parent. There's a wide range of designs, from very basic, no-frills models to the completely tricked-out and Everest-ready. Most people end up happily with something in the middle. "It's not how hard-core the terrain or destination is, but rather, how long you'll be wearing the carrier that determines what model to buy," points out Ann Obenchain, director of marketing at Kelty, a family-oriented outdoor gear company that offers a large line of carriers. "The longer you'll be carrying your child, the more you and your child will appreciate adjustability and comfort features."

More expensive models offer more elaborate suspension systems and more lumbar support. They also tend to have more bells and whistles, such as a weather shield or a hydration system.

BACKPACK BUYING

Here are some guidelines for deciding on what you need:
- If most of your outings are short walks of up to 30 minutes, go with a basic model.
- If you're more likely to go for one to three hours, choose a midrange model with more adjustability and extra gear capacity.
- If you plan on outings of three hours or more, or walks in potentially bad weather, make the investment in a fully loaded, top-of-the-line model, including rain hood and maximum gear capacity.

Cost: $65–$275.

Upside: Lets families explore trails and terrain where strollers can't venture. Allows parents to be active and hands-free with older siblings.

GOOD QUESTION

What essentials should I carry if I take the baby hiking?

One of the delights of parenthood if you enjoy the outdoors is discovering that hiking with young children is surprisingly easy. They tend to be intrigued by the setting, and often spend the time on board drifting between contented sleep and watching the natural world go by.

But hiking with a baby is all the more reason to make sure you're set for the vagaries of the trail. As well as all requisite baby gear (changes of clothes and diapers, wipes, snacks, a favorite toy), lunch, and any nonessentials you bring (camera, binoculars), you should have the following on any hike that will take you more than 20 minutes from the car. We kept a small bag with items 4 through 10 always ready to go—we just quickly checked it (adding the map for our specific locale) before throwing it in the baby backpack and heading out.

1. Water. Enough for the hike, plus an extra bottle.

2. Food. A full lunch, plus some high-energy food (like energy bars and candy) for emergencies.

3. Adverse-conditions gear for the season. In summer, have a hat, sunscreen, and insect repellent.

In spring and fall or if you'll head to higher altitudes, always bring a rain jacket and extra layers for weather worse than you actually expect.

4. First-aid kit. This can be small, but it should include aspirin and acetaminophen, disinfectant wipes, several sizes of Band-Aids, a small and large Ace bandage, some athletic tape, and safety pins.

5. Pocketknife. Not a huge one, but it seems someone always wants an apple cut up or a branch cut off a walking stick.

And if it's a real hike that will take you more than an hour or more than a mile or so from the car, it's worth having the remaining outdoor gear:

6. Lighter. A small piece of candle is nice, too, in case you have to start a fire to dry out wet clothes.

7. Water purification tablets (iodine typically).

8. Whistle. Three loud blasts followed by a break is the universal signal that you're lost or need help.

9. Flashlight and extra batteries. A small light is fine; you may not plan on being out in the dark, but it can be a lifesaver getting you back to the car if you're running late.

10. Compass and map. Be sure the map covers the area well, and learn how to use the compass; try a local outdoor shop for clinics or instructional materials.

Downside: Can be awkward and physically difficult to use (especially with a heavy or older child or for extended periods of time).

Look for these features for baby: A comfortable and adjustable five-point harness; padding on the

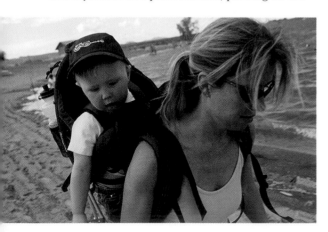

frame, which should also have smooth edges; a seat that spreads baby's legs apart, supports the buttocks, and keeps the knees lower than the buttocks.

Look for these features for you: A comfortable, padded shoulder harness that quickly adjusts for two uses; a padded, adjustable hip belt and lumbar support; a non-finger-pinching kickstand with nonskid feet that opens wide and stable on the ground; easy in and out for baby.

Nice extras: An adjustable cockpit makes it simple to keep your little one comfortable as she grows. Easy-access pockets for keys, diapers, snacks, cell phone, and so on. A toy loop to attach one of baby's favorites; most love a small mirror. Put it on a long string, and you can use it to check on your passenger once in a while.

Brands include: Evenflo, Kelty, REI, Tough Traveler.

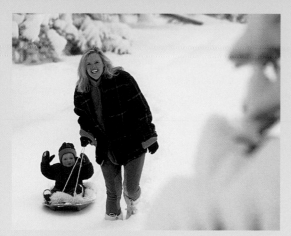

Warming Up to Winter

Dana Kilroy, Reno, Nevada

Dana Kilroy, soon-to-be mother of three, walked through a chilly midwestern winter with her new son Liam (now 6). "No matter how cold it was, I'd bundle him up in fleece buntings with a blanket over him, and keep him close in the Baby Björn so he was warm from my body. I wouldn't go if it was snowing because of the wet, but cold, no problem."

A couple of winters later, when the family had expanded by one and moved to Nevada, Dana and husband Rob snowshoed on weekends, each with a child on their back. "It's important to try different things to find what works," says Dana. "We tried pulling them both in a sled with our snowshoes, but that was just too much work. The backpacks were much easier.

"Even on days when I think it's too cold to be out, my kids are usually game. My daughter grabs a blanket and hops into the jog stroller and my son is willing to layer up and ride his bike, even when it's 38 degrees outside."

PLAY IT SAFE: BACKPACK CARRIERS
The Basics

- Read and follow the manufacturer's directions. Better to take the time and know your gear inside and out than be saying "Hmm, I wonder what this strap is for," and risk an injury.
- Follow the age and weight recommendations.
- Practice putting the backpack carrier on and taking it off several times without baby before his first ride. Do as much adjusting of the harness to fit you before you load your child. The first time you have baby on board (and anytime you think you need it), have someone with you to help you lift the pack and secure it.
- Make sure there's plenty of clearance around you when you lift the pack onto your back. Keep the pack level by lifting from the top at the front and back—the pack can tilt, pitching baby forward.
- Before each use, check the carrier to make sure the straps are all in working order and that nothing is worn or damaged.
- Don't let your child sit or ride in the pack without the harness securely fastened and adjusted.
- Dress your child for the weather, keeping in mind that she won't warm up from motion like you will, and she needs to be protected from the sun.
- Periodically check your child's fit in the carrier. As he grows, you'll need to make adjustments to keep him comfortable.
- Don't use the carrier for activities that compromise your balance—such as skating, bicycling, and downhill skiing.

With Baby on Board

- Regularly check on your passenger (keep a small mirror in your pocket for this) to make sure her position is safe and that she's comfortable. If your child won't ride calmly or stay seated and secure, take her out.
- Be aware that your balance and ability to maneuver will be different with baby riding in the carrier and you take up more space.
- Use extra caution anytime the footing is tricky (mud, ice, or snow-covered surfaces, rocky or root-covered paths) and extra balance is required (stream crossings, steep stairs or slopes, and the like). Consider hiking with one or two poles for added stability.
- Keep an eye out for low-hanging branches, door-ways, and other obstacles that might harm baby.
- Bend your knees (not at the waist) if you need to get low, so that baby isn't hurled forward.
- Don't leave your child in the carrier on any surface other than the ground or floor, and then make sure he's supervised by an adult.

The Art of Diversions; or, Keeping Your Companions Happy on an Outing

Many an outing can be successful so long as your child—no matter what age—is dressed appropriately

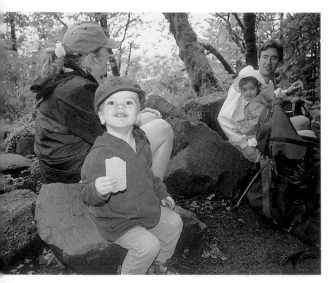

for the weather, given enough to eat and drink, and comfortable. When things turn less than sunny, the next step is to determine whether your little companion is truly tired or uncomfortable, or just bored. If boredom is the culprit, it's handy to have a few tricks up your proverbial sleeve. Cindy Ross and Todd Gladfelter, who spent five summers covering 3,100 miles of wilderness with their two young children, offer these proven strategies from their book *Kids in the Wild: A Family Guide to Outdoor Recreation* (The Mountaineers, 1995), along with a few of our own successful approaches:

Sing. "If I had to pick one thing that helped the most while hiking, it would be singing songs," says Ross. When you can't stand "Itsy Bitsy Spider" anymore, take turns and alternate a children's song with a grown-up tune.

Treasure hunt. Look for deer, ducks, mica, pinecones, flowers, striped rocks, and so on.

Find water. Kids love it in all forms, and it can be a perfect break. When kids get cranky, splash in a creek, look for frogs, build a dam, hunt for shells. Better still, hike to a beach or waterfall.

Break out the toys. Carry a small stash for older babies and present them one by one for maximum mileage. Try regular old stuff, too, like the lid of a baby food jar, a spoon, a small hairbrush, a harmonica.

Teach. Use the opportunity to teach your children about flora and fauna.

Three words: *snacks, snacks, snacks.* You can never have too many nibbles. They can be perfectly healthy and can reenergize even the weariest little legs.

Play games. Try "20 Questions," "I Spy," or make them up. Ross says even her 18-month-old son could join in a game they called "Dog Game." (You name a person or family, and the child responds with the name of their dog.) Older kids might like the "Room Game." (You describe an object in your house, and keep giving clues until the child names the room where the object resides.)

Kids Can Climb Mountains; All You Have to Do Is Ask

Cindy Ross, New Ringgold, Pennsylvania

Not every family is cut out to make big adventure the focus of their lives, but Cindy Ross is living proof that kids and the great outdoors don't have to be mutually exclusive. Ross, an author and adventurer, started her kids early. Very early. While she was six months pregnant with daughter Sierra (now 13), Ross hiked Maine's Mount Katahdin, a 5,268-foot peak at the northern terminus of the Appalachian Trail. "I wanted to do it to celebrate the 10th anniversary of my completion of the trail," she explains. "My husband had to help boost me up near the top where there are iron handholds, because I couldn't quite bend my knees enough, but it wasn't hard. We just took our time."

When she was pregnant with Bryce (now 8), she biked 285 miles on the Chesapeake & Ohio Canal. And when Bryce was 1, the whole family started an epic journey, traveling the 3,100-mile Continental Divide Trail from the Montana–Canada border to the New Mexico–Mexico border, over five summers. "The first summer, we toted 100 cloth diapers, with the assistance of some llama friends," says Ross. "We covered about 9 miles a day when they were little. One and a half hours of hiking, then a one-hour break."

These days the family takes two major trips a year (next up: biking the Yucatán Peninsula, and then later, across Spain, following a 900-year-old pilgrim trail), and fills in the rest of the calendar with plenty of smaller hiking, cycling, and paddling excursions. "At 47, I feel as good as I did when I was 20," says Ross. "And I want to keep moving through my life as I get older. To me, it's more about what you want to do with your life, and walking is a big part of it."

How to Get Wild with Your Kids

If the thought of carrying even a day's worth of diapers plus baby is daunting, take heart. You, too, can take to the trail on the scale of your choice with the following guidance from Cindy Ross:

- Start before your baby is born. "That way, you feel healthy, and walking is already part of your life."
- Do it yourself. "Some women don't have the support of their husbands like I did," acknowledges Ross. "That doesn't mean you can't do it yourself."
- You *can* bring baby. "You stay fit, and she'll be happy, too."
- Start right away. Wait until your child is school age to get started and it may be harder to get him enthused. The younger they start, the more natural the transition from backpack to walker will be. "As four-year-olds my kids could cover 2.5 miles in a hour because they were used to it," says Ross.
- Be willing to adapt. When traditional backpacking was a challenge with small kids, Ross and her husband experimented. They got bikes and a trailer, child carriers, and a canoe–and of course discovered llamas–so that they could still do long trips, just in different formats. A bonus for them: "We found sports that we all love now that we might never have tried otherwise."
- Find your comfort zone. You don't have to vanish into the wilderness for weeks. "Anyone can go camp near their car at a state park," says Ross. "The more you do, the more comfortable you'll feel."
- Remember that kids are resilient. "As long as they were warm, dry, fed, and with us, our kids could deal with almost anything."

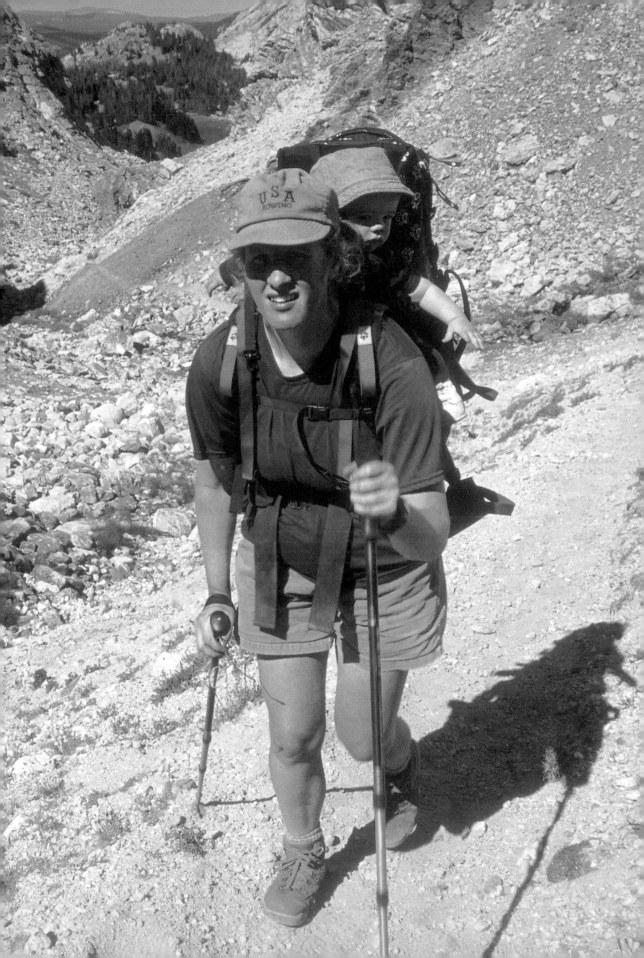

Building a
Balanced Program

18

Boosting the Intensity

Use the Walking Pyramid to start thinking about your goals. Is your focus long-term health, or do you want more? Is working off some baby weight a priority, or do you want to build top aerobic fitness, too? What you want will guide how much of the recommended program you do, and which workouts you make a priority. Use the pyramid as a guide, keeping in mind that the amount of walking is proportional to the size of that section of pyramid.

For *health* and reduced stress levels, 30-minute walks (and some quick stretching afterward) must happen practically every day. That's the broad base of the pyramid.

If *weight loss* is your goal, include four to five longer walks in your week, nudge your speed up a bit (to boost the calorie burn), and be sure to get back to moderate strength training. (A routine is shown in this chapter.) That's the middle of the pyramid.

If complete *fitness* is your goal, add two or three days of shorter, but even faster walks, plus any cross-training for variety. That's the narrow top of the pyramid.

Keep this approach in mind and, come three months from now, you won't be frustrated by pounds that won't seem to budge or still being out of breath at the top of the stairs. You'll be a lean, mean, walking machine.

A Better Build in 20 Minutes a Day

The goals of this straightforward strength training program are to help you rebuild basic muscular fitness and control and to help you get back into a regular habit of resistance exercise. It's a series of total body moves similar to those shown in Trimester II.

The workout is split into an upper- and a lower-body routine. You can do all the exercises at once (it will take about 40 minutes). You can do this two or three times a week.

Or do only one routine at a time; it'll take just 15 to 20 minutes, but you have to do a routine more often—four to six days a week. For example, do the upper-body routine on Monday and Thursday, and the lower-body on Tuesday and Saturday. Consider starting this way for the first few weeks so that you have to carve less time out of your day. Plus, you introduce your muscles to the effort gradually. Then combine them in a total 40-minute routine twice a week; eventually build up to doing the full routine three times a week.

However you break it up (two or four days a week), do the exercises in the order shown, and do two sets of 12 repetitions with only a short break in between, unless stated otherwise.

The Walking Pyramid

GOAL: HOW MUCH WALKING? HOW OFTEN?
INTENSITY: HOW HARD TO WORK? HEART RATE;
RATE OF PERCEIVED EXERTION; SPEED

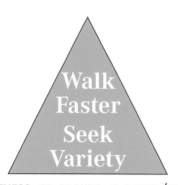

Walk Faster Seek Variety

FITNESS 20-30 MINS. 2-3 DAYS/WK.
INTENSITY: 75%-90% OF MAX. HR, RPE: 7-9, 4.0+ MPH

Walk Longer Build Strength

WEIGHT LOSS 45-60+ MINS. 4-5 DAYS/WK.
INTENSITY: 60%-75% OF MAX. HR, RPE: 5-7, 3.5-4.0 MPH

Walk Daily Stretch Often

HEALTH 30+ MINUTES 6+ DAYS/WK.
INTENSITY: 50%-65% OF MAX. HR, RPE: 4-6, 3.0-3.5 MPH

Begin at the bottom of the pyramid and work your way up, balancing type and intensity of walk.

What Do You Need?

The program is displayed in terms of using your own body weight, a floor mat, free weights, and a simple bench. With a set of 3- to 15-pound dumbbells, just about anyone should be able to do the program just about anywhere.

If you go to a club or gym and prefer to use machines, you can simply replicate the moves described here. But using free weights for at least some of the moves can help improve balance and coordination while building strength.

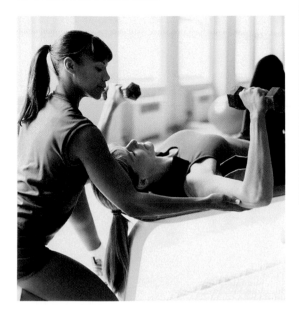

1 **Chest press.** Lie on your back on a bench, with weights in your hands at your shoulders. Slowly press your arms all the way out to fully extended, then back down.

2 **Bent-over row.** Begin with your right hand and knee on a bench, left foot on the floor, left arm hanging down with the weight, back flat and parallel to ground. Slowly pull the weight up to your shoulder, squeezing your shoulder blades to finish; slowly return to start. Repeat the set on other side.

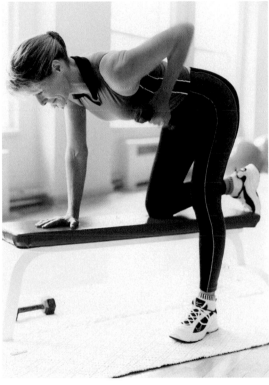

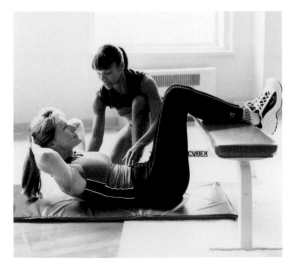

3 **Abdominal crunch.** Lie on your back with knees bent, feet on the ground, arms crossed, and hands on opposite shoulders. Look at the ceiling to keep your neck relaxed; slowly contract your abdominal muscles to lift your shoulders off the floor; hold the crunch for a two-count, then relax. Start with 12, but build up to 20 repetitions. **To increase resistance:** First move your hands up next to your ears, elbows out to the sides. Second, place your feet up on a bench or sofa.

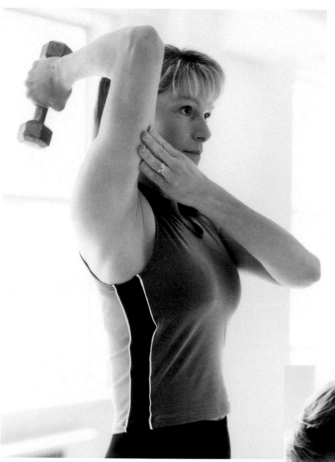

4 **Triceps extension.** Point the elbow of your right arm toward the ceiling with the elbow bent, forearm down, and hand holding a weight behind your right shoulder. Steady the right elbow with your left hand. Slowly straighten the right arm; fully extend but don't lock the elbow, then return to the start position.

Lift Right (Then Left): Five Tips for Effective, Safe Weight Lifting

1. Concentrate on good, slow technique—don't let momentum do the work for you—and move your joints through their full range of motion.

2. When possible, exhale while lifting the weight, inhaling on the recovery or between reps.

3. Maintain good posture. Focus on stabilizing your body throughout all movements with the abdominal and back muscles.

4. Lifting shouldn't hurt, but it should be hard. Select a weight so that you're just able to finish the designated number of repetitions on the last set but would be hard pressed to do more.

5. Keep progressing. When a weight becomes easy to lift, add more. Increase to the next weight and reduce the number of repetitions if necessary, until you're able to build up to the full target number again.

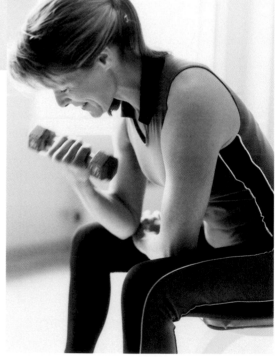

5 **Biceps curl.** Seated on a bench with legs spread, place your right elbow on the right knee, braced with the left hand. Your right hand holds the weight, and the arm starts straight—slowly bend it until the weight is up at the shoulder, then return to the start position.

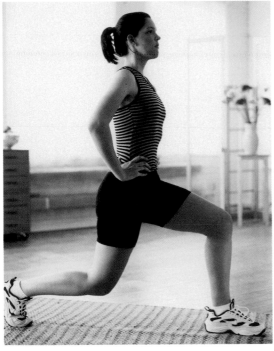

LOWER-BODY ROUTINE

1 **Abdominal crunch.** Same as the upper-body routine.

2 **Lunge.** Start with both feet together. Take a giant step forward while bending your forward knee (maintain a tall posture; don't push your bending knee beyond the foot). Then press forcefully off your forward leg to return to standing. Alternate 10 reps on each leg.
To increase resistance: Hold light dumbbells.

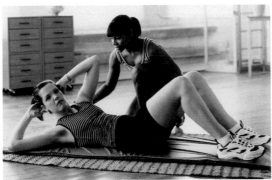

3 **Side crunch.** Start like abdominal crunches: lying on your back with knees bent, feet on the ground, arms crossed, and hands on opposite shoulders. Look at the ceiling to keep your neck relaxed; slowly contract your abdominal muscles to lift your right shoulder off the floor, twisting so the right elbow goes toward the left knee. Relax. Do 12 reps in each direction.
To increase resistance: First move your hands up next to your ears, elbows out to the sides. Second, place your feet up on a bench or sofa.

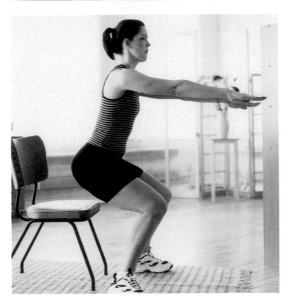

4 **Squat.** Stand tall, with your feet hip width apart, hands at your sides or arms extended for balance. Bend your knees and hips to slowly drop to a half-sitting position, keeping your upper body as erect as possible, then stand back up. Do 15 reps; if this isn't tiring, hold light dumbbells.

5 **Alternate arm/leg extension.** Begin on your hands and knees on the floor, with your head level and back flat. Extend your right arm and left leg out straight, parallel to ground. Hold for five seconds, then drop; repeat on the other side. Begin with 6 reps on each side, build to 12 on each side. (See chapter 15 for a photo.)

Pushing off
with your
back foot and
extending
your toes
behind you
builds speed
and shapely
calf muscles.

The Walking Program, Postmester III

Now that your life with the baby is settling somewhat—consistent eating and sleeping patterns, with her looking forward to your daily walks—you can build more variety into your exercise. It's time to explore all the different ways you can build walking into your life: brief but speedy walks when time is short, long rambles when you have time to explore, and functional walks built into your day whenever the destination is close enough. This mix will make it hard to get bored, and help you build walking as a lifetime habit.

GENERAL REMINDERS FOR POSTMESTER III

- Walk somewhere. Whenever you can, take a walk in lieu of a ride in the car. Or do "trip-chaining": Park in one place, bring along a stroller or backpack, and you and baby walk to several destinations at once, building your walking into something you have to do anyway.
- Pick up the pace. You should be fully healed from the rigors of pregnancy, so unless the doctor has urged you to hold back, get your walking tempo back in gear. Get all your walks back to a healthy, moderate tempo (more than 3.0 mph), but at least twice a week try to put a little speed on. The programs recommend either a "B" for brisk pace (3.5 to 4.0 mph) or an "F" for a fast tempo (more than 4.0 mph) for several walks a week. Warm up and cool down at an easy pace for the first and last five minutes of the walk; pick up the speed for the remainder in the middle.
- Boost your walking time. You and the baby are a walking team by now. So make a team effort to keep pushing your walking time up, adding five minutes to your longer walks every week.
- Stick with the basics. Warm up briefly before every walk. Stretch every day, either the quick stretches or the full stretch routine; by now you know what your body needs just by how you feel.
- Get strong again. At the very least keep up the core strength routine, but ideally add the full strength routine (shown in this chapter) two or more times a week.

LOW-KEY PROGRAM, POSTMESTER III

WEEKLY GOALS FOR THE LOW-KEY PROGRAM

- Shoot for a total of 180 minutes of walking a week. At an average of six 30-minute walks a week, this meets the surgeon general's recommendation for long-term health.

- At least four days a week, walk at least 30 minutes, even if it's broken up. Get up to 40 minutes for at least one walk a week, if not more.

- Pick up the pace on two of your weekly walks. Go easy for the first 5 minutes, speed up for the middle 10 to 15 minutes, then cool down for the last 5 minutes. Target a brisk pace for the quick part. For many women, that's 3.5 to 4.0 mph, or an RPE of 5 to 7 on the 10-point scale.

- Do the quick stretches after every walk. Twice a week, try to make it the full stretch routine (not shown in the sample week).

- Do the core routine (five exercises) at least four days a week. When you feel ready, convert one or two of these weekly workouts to the full strength routine shown in this chapter.

A TYPICAL WEEK NEAR THE END OF POSTMESTER III, LOW-KEY PROGRAM:							
	MON.	TUES.	WED.	THUR.	FRI.	SAT.	SUN.
WALK (minutes)	25 (B)	35	20, 10	30 (B)	20	40	OFF
OTHER STUFF	CORE	CORE	CORE		CORE	CORE	

"B" is a brisk walk, 3.5–4.0 mph or more.

MODERATE PROGRAM, POSTMESTER III

WEEKLY GOALS FOR THE MODERATE PROGRAM

▪ Target a total of about 225 minutes of walking a week—that means you're exceeding an average of six days of walking at least 35 minutes a day.

▪ At least four days a week, shoot for 30 minutes of walking, even if it's broken up. On a fifth day, try for a 45-minute walk or more.

▪ Pick up the pace on two of your weekly walks. Go easy for the first 5 to 10 minutes, speed up for the middle 20 to 25 minutes, then cool down for the last 5 minutes. Target a brisk pace (for many women, that's 3.5 to 4.0 mph, or an RPE of 5 to 7 on the 10-point scale) for the speedy part.

▪ Do the quick stretches after every walk; several days when you feel you need it, make it the full stretch routine (not shown in the program).

▪ Get stronger. Do the full strength routine (shown this chapter) at least twice a week, and the short core strength routine two or three other days. Or split the strength routine in half and do it four days a week.

A TYPICAL WEEK NEAR THE END OF POSTMESTER III, MODERATE PROGRAM:						
	MON.	**TUES.**	**WED.**	**THUR.**	**FRI.**	**SAT.**	**SUN.**
WALK (minutes)	35 (B)	45	35	40 (B)	20 (B)	50	OFF
OTHER STUFF	CORE	FULL STRENGTH	CORE		FULL STRENGTH	CORE	

"B" is a brisk walk, 3.5–4.0 mph or more.

CHALLENGING PROGRAM, POSTMESTER III

WEEKLY GOALS FOR THE CHALLENGING PROGRAM

▪ At a total of about 250 minutes of walking a week, you're averaging more than 40 minutes a day for six days of walking. This is a healthy dose of walking, especially as you pick up the pace.

▪ Shoot for several 30- to 45-minute walks, another of 50 minutes, and at least one weekly walk of an hour by the end of this postmester.

▪ Pick up the pace on at least two weekly walks. Walk easy for the first 5 to 10 minutes, pick it up for the middle 20 to 25 minutes, then cool down for the last 5 minutes. Target a brisk pace (RPE of 5 to 7) for one walk, go downright fast (RPE of 7 to 9) for the other.

▪ Keep stretching daily. Do the quick stretches every day, or replace them with the full stretches whenever you feel a tight spot coming on.

▪ Get strong again. Do the full strength routine (shown this chapter) three days of the week, and the core routine two or three more days.

A TYPICAL WEEK NEAR THE END OF POSTMESTER III, CHALLENGING PROGRAM:							
	MON.	**TUES.**	**WED.**	**THUR.**	**FRI.**	**SAT.**	**SUN.**
WALK (minutes)	35 (F)	50	30 (B)	45	30	60	OFF
OTHER STUFF	FULL STRENGTH	CORE	FULL STRENGTH	CORE	FULL STRENGTH	CORE	

"B" is a brisk walk, 3.5–4.0 mph or more; "F" is fast, better than 4.0 mph at the least.

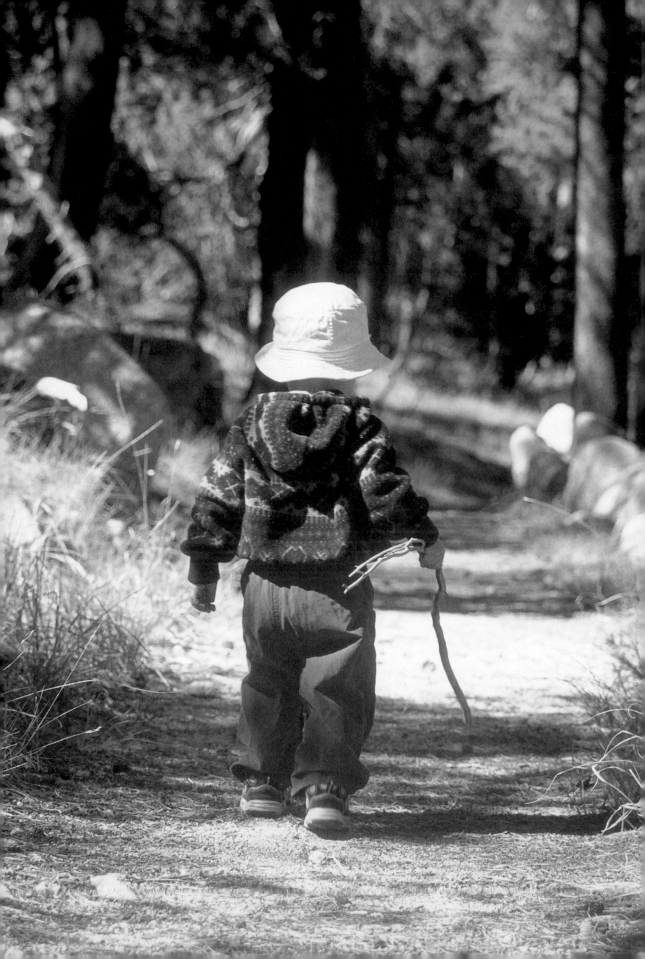

A Lifetime of Physical Activity

19

What Matters to Moms

One idea came up again and again in our discussions with pregnant women and new mothers. And it isn't what you might expect. It wasn't that everyone had a perfect pregnancy or delivery just because they were fit. Babies came early and late, naturally and by Cesarean. It wasn't that they all found it easy to exercise. Older children, jobs, moving, being a single parent all made exercise during and after pregnancy a real challenge. And it's not that they were all superathletes for whom pregnancy was just a little bump in the road. Sure, Evan Garner wanted to keep her maximal fitness so she could go right back to marathon training after the baby was born. But Sue Ryder was pregnant with twins, trying not to be lapped by 80-year-olds at the community center track and struggling to keep from tipping the scales with a 50-pound weight gain.

No, the thread that tied them all together was much simpler: Walking was, or had become, a way of life. Even if they weren't avid walkers before pregnancy, all realized the elegant simplicity of walking as the ideal exercise choice both while pregnant and after. What's more, almost all spoke of building walking into their lives. For many, walking for errands and routine daily tasks was one way they made sure they'd get their daily fix. And it wasn't just when walking was convenient; everyone we spoke to tried to build walking into every day.

That leads to the final question of this book, the most important question. And that question is not whether *you* will continue to be a walker, but rather . . .

WILL YOUR CHILD BE A WALKER?

At about nine months of age, your child is largely dependent on you for mobility. You tote him to the mailbox and back. Boost him into the backpack to go grocery shopping. Strap him into the jogging stroller to walk the dog. But soon, he will discover that his feet can do more than kick off his booties. He'll take those first steps and transition from passenger to pedestrian. You've laid the proper groundwork by showing your child that walking is an important part of daily life. And the time you spend together walking and exploring now and in his early years can make the difference between starting your child on the road to becoming a healthy, active adult or consigning him to join the growing ranks of overweight, sedentary Americans.

The obesity epidemic is not just a grown-up problem. According to the National Institutes of Health, 15 percent of American children are severely overweight (essentially obese). That's three times as many as 30 years ago.

TIP:

Speed tips: Walk tall, shoulders back, gaze forward, focus on faster (not longer) steps and quick, compact arm swings.

A recent survey that compared activity levels among schoolchildren in three countries provides an alarming snapshot of the situation. When researchers studied children in the United States, Australia, and Sweden, they found American kids on the bottom rung when it comes to physical activity. American boys were 20 percent less active than boys in Sweden, and 10 percent less active than those in Australia. American girls were on par with Australian girls but, like the boys, 20 percent less active than Swedish girls. Not surprisingly, the American children in the study were roughly twice as likely to be overweight. "This study clearly tells us that even among very young children, physical activity provides a critical barrier to obesity," says Robert P. Pangrazi, PhD, one of the researchers on the study and a professor at Arizona State University.

"It's a huge problem," says Melvin B. Heyman, MD, MPH, professor of pediatrics and chief of pediatric gastroenterology, hepatology, and nutrition at the University of California, San Francisco. "These children are likely to grow up to be overweight adults. Whether or not their health is affected as children, they'll definitely be affected psychosocially, and they are at risk for developing diabetes or other complications. When you're talking about that large a percentage of the population, the impact on society, the economy, and the health care industry over the years will be tremendous."

By being active with your child, you tackle many of the central issues surrounding childhood overweight head-on. "The two biggest factors are a lack of activity, plus a combination of eating the wrong foods and lack of portion control," says Heyman. If you're active, it sets a healthy example (see "Role Call") and gives your child less opportunity to nest on the couch.

"Active parents tend to have active children," he adds. "If parents are on the go, it not only encourages the children, it also gives them less time to sit around." Active parents also are more likely to control their own weight, which is another risk factor for kids. "The risk is greater for the child to be overweight if one parent is overweight, and much greater if both parents are overweight."

Next, consider that habits—healthy or otherwise—start in infancy. As soon as babies start eating, they get messages that stick about portion size (how much oatmeal or how many crackers you offer). They learn whether a treat means a sugary cookie or fresh blueberries. No wonder, then, that the older the overweight child is, the harder it will be for him to gain control of his weight. Overweight adolescents have a 70 percent chance of becoming overweight or obese adults.

How Big Is Baby, Postmester IV (10 months and up)?

At ten months of age, baby now weighs between 15 and 24 pounds. At this point, the rate at which she gains tends to slow somewhat, but still continues to steadily rise.

Key milestones: Baby's day follows a predictable schedule. At about nine months, depth perception develops, making the view from the backpack even more interesting for baby. Her distance vision advances greatly between ages 1 and 2. Most babies are crawling and pull up to standing. Most start walking a month or two after their first birthday, but first steps could come substantially earlier or later.

What this means for you: Baby enjoys backpack and stroller rides even more, but you may have to plan outings more carefully to avoid interfering with nap or bedtime. Once baby is mobile—crawling, pulling up, toddling—she'll probably appreciate time to move around on her own before you plunk her in a carrier or stroller for a walk (particularly if she's just been strapped into the high chair or car seat). On longer outings, bring drinks, snacks, and a toy or two.

GOOD QUESTION

How do we move from my child riding to walking?

Already, your 9- to 12-month old may be scrambling to get out of the stroller, and he'll be moving under his own power in no time (if not already!). So how best to make it easy on both the baby and you? Cindy Ross, author of four books on outdoor adventures with kids, was exploring the wilderness with her two children from the time they were babies in backpack carriers. Your perambulations may be on a smaller scale, but you'll still appreciate Ross's advice on how to manage this transition.

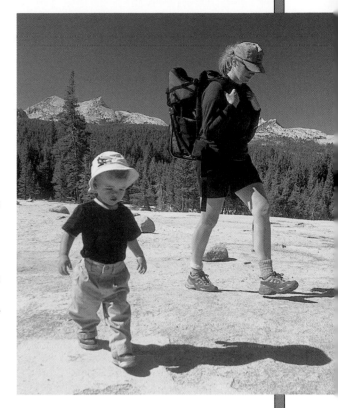

- **The difficult years.** Ages 1 to 3 is the toughest, says Ross, because your child is too young to walk too far and too heavy to be carried for any distance. Expect to do a lot of in and out of the backpack. Choose walks with lots of long, easy stretches where little ones can get out and explore. Pick walks with diversions, such as a flat, streamside trail that ends up at a lake.

- **Weaning from the backpack.** Tote the carrier, even though you might not use it. Encourage your children to walk, but don't force them if they resist. When they're too heavy to carry, choose short walks and hikes and leave the pack at home.

- **How far?** First, choose according to the youngest in the group. Most four-year-olds can handle 2 miles if they're fit and used to outings. But it's not just the distance that counts. Consider where you're walking and alter your plan accordingly. Is it flat sidewalk? Gently sloping? Up and down? Steep? Smooth path? Rocky or root-covered trail? And of course, the weather. If it's hot, cold, rainy, or windy, you need to adjust.

- **Cheerlead.** Encourage—but don't push—your children to walk whenever they seem interested. At first, this will slow you down a great deal, but it will be worth it in the long run. Tell them they are great hikers whenever things are going well and at the end of every outing.

- **Outfit them.** Kids love to have the same stuff that you do. Outfitting them with a small backpack filled with a snack, sunglasses and hat, and a stuffed animal is a great motivator. Sometimes we do this even just for an extended shopping walk downtown.

- **Be sensitive.** Kids not only move at a slower pace, they also live in the moment. That means your goal—reaching a summit or outlook—doesn't hold the same allure for them. If they just want to stop and scramble on rocks at trailside, maybe that's the best thing to do.

- **Keep track.** Preschoolers and grade schoolers love to tally and review their achievements. Make a book together that records major family walks and hikes. Have the kids paste in photos. This helps underscore their achievement, and gives them something to look back on—maybe before the next big adventure—and say, "Hey, I did that!"

Bottom Line: It's fantastic to watch your child go from a passenger to a walker, and you can help her enjoy every step. The key is to be flexible, adjust your expectations, and enjoy the little things. Allow your child to set the tempo and have positive walking experiences, and you're guaranteed to be raising a walker for life.

GOOD QUESTION

What "things" in your life help you maintain an active lifestyle with kids?

A survey of our active families offered a range of ideas from costly hardware to clever habits.

- "Without a doubt the double jogger that the family all pitched in and bought for us. I use it every day, sometimes twice a day, now that the girls are big enough. I would be a crazy woman without it! How else can you walk or run with twins?"

- "Loud music and dancing with the kids."

- "Having a dog makes us get out and walk or run. We walk the abandoned rail corridor during the fall, winter, and spring. It always makes us feel better to get outside for at least one outing a day!"

- "Binoculars, because for kids to be able to really see something at a distance is to want to go there."

- "Having a treadmill in my house is the key to me getting any exercise at all because, in theory any- way, I can get on it at funky times; when the child(ren) are napping, at five o'clock in the morn- ing, or after they go to bed at night."

- "Walks to the beach. No way you can go there and not want to dig and bury and splash and run around and look for stuff and throw little rocks and climb on big ones. It's the perfect outdoor gym."

- "A baby backpack. It's great for places that aren't stroller-friendly; a walk in the woods, a tour around a farm, berry picking. I remember having Molly in that thing and passing berries back to her to eat and whoa, what a vision her little smeared face was when I finally got her out."

- "Our fire pit. Great for family marshmallow roasts after a walk . . ."

- "My sister thoughtfully picked out a Baby Jogger for me so that I could continue to get my exercise. This is truly my favorite possession!"

- "The promise of a warm-weather vacation two months after giving birth to David; we all (but espe- cially I) wanted to be in shape to walk the beach!"

Bottom Line: Sure, you need the hardware—front carriers, strollers, backpacks for babies, maybe a treadmill or dog for you. But it's clear these folks had an attitude that activity was a priority, and they were going to make it happen—and have fun, too.

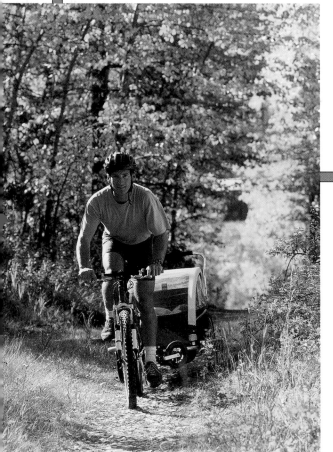

Even without considering changes in diet, being active can have an impact. "Even if you don't change your diet a bit, taking the stairs versus the escalator every day makes a difference of sev- eral pounds a year," points out Heyman.

Even the experts admit this is no easy task. Heyman—also a parent who faces the challenges of television, computer, and cars that all make it easier for kids to sit than move—is the first to admit this. But by at least being aware of the challenges to being active, you stand a fighting chance to create opportunities to get your child moving.

Role Call: Kids Take Cues from Active Parents

Compelling research continues to emerge, under-lining how vital it is for Mom and Dad to both walk the talk about being active and encourage their children to choose tag over Nintendo, soccer over Cyberchase.

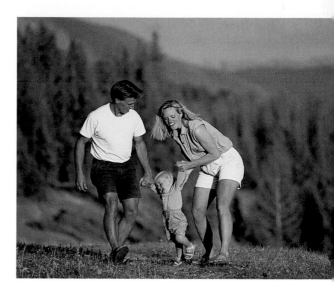

This is particularly important for parents of girls, who tend to be less active than boys, and are also more influenced by their parents. One recent study of 180 nine-year-old girls and their parents found that although dads are more often active themselves, and thus provide a positive role model, the logistics that moms typically take care of (sign-ups, taxiing, spectating) are just as effective in getting girls moving. Here's how powerful parental involvement was:

- When neither parent gave support, less than 30 percent of the girls were highly active.
- When one parent gave support, 56 percent of the girls were highly active.
- When both parents gave support, 70 percent were highly active.

"These results send a clear message to parents that they can play a key role in promoting physical activity among their children," says Kirsten Krahnstoever Davison, PhD, lead author of the Pennsylvania State University study. "Support from one parent is likely to have a positive impact, and support from both parents is even better." Exactly how young does support count? Researchers don't exactly know. "But I would speculate that this modeling effect occurs quite young," adds Davison. "Being a positive role model is appropriate at any age."

She offers these age-related guidelines on promoting active kids:

- **Babies.** Be active yourself, and take baby along.
- **Toddlers.** Allow toddlers to move freely. Limit time in swings, high chairs, and playpens. Make sure your home and yard are safe for your child to explore.
- **Young children.** Take them to playgrounds and get them outside to play with supervision as much as possible. Include them in family walks, hikes, and bike rides, and make sure kids use their own power, instead of hitching a ride. When kids are physically and emotionally ready, try community-based sports and activities that emphasize fun, not competition.

Your Community Matters to Your Child's Health

Striking research was published in two special issues of research journals regarding America's epidemic of sedentary living. The September 2003 issues of both the *American Journal of Public Health* and *American Journal of Health Promotion* focused on a single question: Can your environment determine whether you're physically active? Or more simply, can where you live actually make you fat? And the compelling answer gleaned from many of the articles was, "Yes!"

❊**TIP:**

Take stairs instead of elevators whenever you can. Make a walk part of your commute once a week. Ride mass transit? Get off a stop early!

GOOD QUESTION

Why don't kids walk to school anymore?

The Centers for Disease Control is so concerned about the epidemic of childhood obesity that it's been doing research into this question. It found that many parents reported the distance was too great or that weather was a barrier. The first is likely related to the tremendous consolidation of schools nationwide, and elimination of neighborhood schools—a trend some communities are now reexamining, in part because of the great cost of transporting all the students by bus. Other concerns were dangerous traffic and the fear of crime.

Communities all over the country are responding to

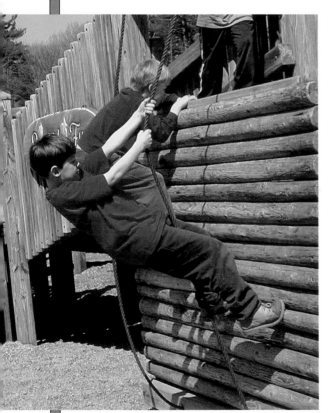

these concerns by launching creative programs to encourage more walking and cycling to school. Often called "Safe Routes to School," they include measures to slow traffic near schools, repair or build missing sidewalks, improve street crossings and hire crossing guards, teach pedestrian safety to kids, and

even reestablish neighborhood schools! One unique approach: Launch walking school buses, which are groups of kids walking a route to school with designated adults (usually parent volunteers), picking up kids along the way. Authors Mark and Lisa lead one every day, and the success of such efforts even in northern climates proves that kids are not necessarily softer than they were 25 years ago, when far more kids did walk to school; they've simply gotten in the habit of being chauffeured everywhere.

But why is it so great for a child to be able to walk or bicycle to school? Here are just a few reasons:

- Improved health. The obvious one—physically active children are at reduced risk for obesity and a slew of related physical and emotional concerns.

- Improved academic performance. Children who are more fit did better in school than those with low fitness in a recent California study; in part researchers credit better attention spans.

- Better discipline. Teachers report that kids who've gotten exercise in the morning are more calm and ready to work.

- Improved air quality. The EPA reports measurably better air quality around schools where more of the students walk and bike. Schools with lots of parents shuttling kids in cars have dramatically worse air quality at drop-off and pickup times— exactly when children are outside the school in that cloud of fumes.

- Better navigational skills and social development. British researchers (where they've been studying this longer) fear that kids who are driven everywhere never learn how to find their own way, and lack the skills to recognize dangerous situations because they're never out and about on foot.

- Better drivers? Not proven, but it's thought that kids who walk and are taught to cross streets safely learn to estimate the speed and distance of oncoming cars; those who spend life in the back of a mini van never practice such skills until driving age, which is much too late.

- It's more fun. Kids love to be able to get out of the car or bus and spend that time unconstrained and walking with friends—it's what kids are meant to do.

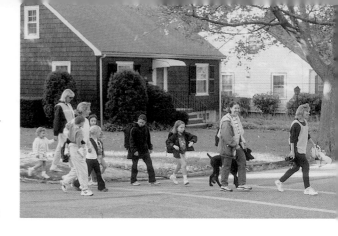

A number of studies showed that people who lived in more sprawling, less walkable settings were in fact likely to walk less and actually be heavier. That's even taking into account such factors as income and educational level, which are known to affect how much people exercise. (Wealthier, more educated households tend to exercise more.)

A number of attributes were found to relate to how likely it is that people walk in an area. Most confirm what you'd already suspect:

- **Sidewalks.** Communities with more connected, comprehensive sidewalk networks have more walking. Shorter blocks and street grids (as you'd see in a traditional downtown) give pedestrians more choices and better connections.
- **Parks and bike trails.** Both are ideal walking destinations, and are known to increase walking in the area. Many longer trails are becoming bike and pedestrian commuter highways, while smaller "pocket" parks are ideal neighborhood destinations for families.
- **Compact neighborhoods.** Building on smaller lots means distances between destinations are shorter and more walkable. Modern sprawling developments—one-acre and larger housing lots, massive shopping complexes—create distances that are just too far for most people to walk.
- **Mixed uses.** If homes, shopping, schools, worksites, and recreational opportunities are all intermingled, it's easy to live within walking distance of where you want to go during the day. But once you separate the uses—housing subdivisions over here, office parks there, strip malls and big-box stores in another place—every trip has to be by car. The worst offense: consolidated schools on the periphery of town where land is cheap (lower taxes) and every child has to be bussed or driven.
- **Ample mass transit.** Reliable bus, subway, and light rail service all help; they're only likely in more developed settings, but important because most transit trips start and end with a walk or bike trip. (Many city buses now even carry bike racks up front to encourage cycling.)

- **Calmer traffic.** Slow down the cars and make it easier to cross streets, and people will walk more. Done right, it can also help to smooth rather than restrict traffic flows.
- **Safety.** The threat of crime will keep people—especially children—inside. But what's one of the most effective ways to improve personal security? Simply get more people out on the street—that's what makes walkers feel safe.
- **People-friendly architecture.** Houses facing the street with front porches, and storefronts near the sidewalk with lots of windows, are welcoming to pedestrians, making passersby feel safe. But build a big concrete box surrounded by acres of asphalt parking, and you can be sure that everyone will be showing up by car, not on foot.

YEAH, BUT WHAT CAN I DO ABOUT IT?

And what about *you*? Quite simply, helping to create a more walkable, livable community may be one of the most lasting gifts you can give your child. So get involved personally. Many of the decisions that affect the walkability of your community—transportation and land-use planning—are made at the local level, where a small number of vocal citizens can have a huge impact. Work through the following four levels.

1. Be a Role Model

You've already started by being a regular walker. But maybe you can establish a new norm for your neighborhood by forgoing at least one car trip every day, and biking or walking with your child instead. As your child gets older, walk to day

GOOD QUESTION

Where do I take my child to interest her in walking?

Our panel of moms offered lots of insights on the best places to walk with young children—particularly when the child is ready to start exploring, too.

- "My favorite trip was when we'd meet a friend and her son and walk up the bike path to the library for a sing-along. It was my favorite part of the week— a combo of exercise, social time, and baby time."

- "Walking to the Museum of Science or the Museum of Fine Arts in Boston—lots of things for both of us to see in such rich, visual places."

- "Any place that involved ponds, ducks, geese, and walking."

- "We got a membership at the zoo and visited almost once a week, in all but the coldest weather. Sometimes it was just for the walk there and back—with the membership, we didn't feel we had to stay past my daughter's interest just to get our money's worth; we'd be back next week."

- "The playground. It was baby-social central, the perfect place to network with other moms and develop play groups. It was also great to observe other babies and their parents, and learn that my kids were normal and I wasn't crazy after all."

- "In Chicago, we could walk to go see the train go by—entertainment in itself."

- "Local conservation land with glacial erratics—the refrigerator- to VW-sized rocks left by glaciers—all along the trail. Those forming a pile just perfect for the kids to scramble on have become known as the "snack" rocks, for obvious reasons."

This, from our editor Ann at The Lyons Press, caught themes that were repeated again and again by parents we spoke to:

- "Susie insists on walking on the trails now, and goes crazy for wooden boardwalks over rocky areas and streams. She likes to walk back and forth, back and forth and, to torture mommy, peer over the edge. It makes for a slower walk, but I can't hurry her along—she pitches a fit if I try to rush her."

Bottom Line: Although baby oriented settings—playgrounds, parks, and library story-hours—are common targets, a surprising number of parents and children find great entertainment in the mundane. A local duck pond, rail crossing, or trail with a footbridge or climbable rocks can provide a perfectly delightful target, especially as it becomes familiar and your child looks forward to getting there. Parents also offered that "grown up" destinations, such as museums and arboretums, can be just as visually stimulating to young explorers.

---

care, school, soccer, and band practice. Even better, co-opt your friends. When the kids want a play date, don't drive and drop her off in the car; instead, agree with the other parent to walk and meet halfway, transferring the kids there. Or you walk them over, and he or she walks them back.

2. Be a Lone Voice

Show up at planning and zoning meetings, ask questions, and at least make people explain why it's being done the way it is. Here's the shocking thing—sometimes a small handful of people showing up at a meeting and asking for a change can affect the outcome of a key decision, such as whether a new subdivision has sidewalks or a playground, or whether a new store devotes more space to parking or to making safe pedestrian access and a useful bike parking area.

3. Infiltrate Existing Entities

Mark ran for the local planning board and found that nothing is as effective as being on the "inside." If all he does is get the sidewalk network closer to completion in the community, it will be time well spent. But you can have an impact working on all of the following and many others:

- **Planning or zoning board.** Drive more compact and thoughtful land-use decisions and fight the sprawl that is so discouraging to daily walking.

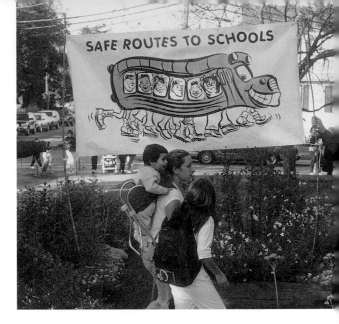

- **School board.** Help get a walk-and-bike-to-school program launched; get pedestrian and bicycle safety curricula put in place.
- **Town or city council.** Everything from funding sidewalk construction to the school budget affect whether your child will have a place to walk.
- **Recreation or conservation commissions.** Trails and greenways, playing fields and parks are all critical to living an active life.
- **Neighborhood association.** Slowing the traffic, getting a sidewalk on your street, and keeping it clear and well maintained is a great place to start.

4. Create a New Coalition

Get others involved, and make people in different disciplines talk to one another. Is your planning board working with your school board? Is the department of public works connected to the health department? Some of the best solutions come from these kinds of collaborations. A great starting point is getting a simple neighborhood walkability checklist in the hands of residents, so they become aware of why they do or don't walk. In many cities and towns, this has led to the creation of a standing "walkable community committee" (see the "Good Question" box). Eventually, your group could launch a neighborhood safety campaign, a community traffic calming project, a walk-to-school program, or something similar.

GOOD QUESTION

Whom should we invite to be on our walkable community committee? What should we do?

Here's a starter list of people to invite to take part in the effort to make your community more friendly to walking. Surprisingly, many of these people may be thinking about the same issues, and will be delighted to hook up with others who care about making your town more livable. Start with a discussion of all your favorite places in town, and your least favorites. Then start thinking about what could make bad spots more like the good ones!

- Health departments.
- Police, fire, public safety.
- Departments of public works and transportation engineering.
- Planning, zoning, and land-use officials.

- Chambers of commerce, downtown or small-business associations.
- School committees or superintendents.
- Parks, recreation departments, conservation and open-space committees.
- Neighborhood associations and any interested citizens.
- Bicycle or pedestrian advocacy organizations (there are hundreds of these around the country).
- Elected officials and their staffs (mayor, county executive, city or county council members, local legislators).

Bottom Line: It takes cooperation among lots of professional entities to make your community more livable and walkable. But most important to the process can be the regular citizens who add energy, common sense, and a drive for positive change.

NEIGHBORHOOD WALKABILITY CHECKLIST

(Adapted from the checklist of the Partnership for a Walkable America; www.walkinginfo.org)

Take this checklist on a typical walk (to a friend's house, your child's day care, the corner store) and share copies with friends. Note things that might discourage you (and a child) from walking regularly and their locations. Score each from 1 through 6; compare notes to identify the biggest problems. Then talk to public officials and set priorities for making improvements.

1. Did you have room to walk?
(6—room for 2 or 3 people; 1—barely enough for 1)
Score: ___
___ Yes.
___ No. Common problems:
No sidewalks or broken ones; sidewalks blocked with poles, signs, Dumpsters; no paths or trails; no shoulders.
Comments, locations:_____
_____
_____

2. Was it easy to cross streets?
(6—no problem; 1—it took forever and was scary)
Score: ___
___ Yes.
___ No. Common problems:
Roads too wide to get across; signals made us wait too long, or didn't give enough crossing time; needed striped crosswalks or traffic signals; parked cars, trees, or other things blocked our view of traffic; needed curb ramps.
Comments, locations:_____
_____
_____

3. Was it a pleasant place to walk?
(6—I'd love to go back; 1—no reason to be there)
Score: ___
___ Yes.
___ No. Common problems:
Needs more grass, flowers, or trees, water fountains, shade, benches; too dark, dirty; no art, natural, architectural, or historic features. Few desirable destinations (stores, restaurants, a library, post office, schools, bus or subway stops).
Comments, locations:_____
_____
_____

4. Was traffic a problem?
(6—didn't notice it; 1—lots of cars, too fast, too close)
Score: ___
___ No.
___ Yes. Common problems:
There were too many cars, or traffic was too fast. Drivers backed out of driveways without looking; did not yield to pedestrians; turned toward people crossing side streets; drove too fast; sped up to get through traffic lights; stopped in or blocked crosswalks.
Comments, locations:_____
_____
_____

5. Did you feel safe?
(6—I'd walk alone, anytime; 1—scary, even with others in daylight)
Score: ___
___ Yes.
___ No. Common problems:
Saw suspicious activity or people; no apparent houses, stores, or other places to go in case of trouble; no public telephones; too dark; too few other pedestrians—too little activity on the street.
Comments, locations:_____
_____
_____

CHECK YOUR SCORE:

26–30: Terrific. You live in a great walking community.

21–25: Good. But focus on trouble spots.

16–20: Fair. Get your neighbors and elected officials involved immediately.

15 or less: Call out the national guard—it's no fun walking there, and it needs work.

MAKING THE WORLD MORE WALKABLE

If your walking route scored poorly, then take action. Share your findings with elected officials (for example, the mayor's office or city council) and public services. Start with the department of public works, transportation, and police departments. Let them—and the media—know about specific trouble spots. Also, get out and fix what you can. Here are some simple things you can do; urge family and friends to join your efforts:

DO IT YOURSELF

- **Select better, safer routes** to walk if necessary. But that's not enough!
- **Trim hedges or trees** that block sidewalks or the view at a crosswalk.
- **Plant beautifying trees and flowers** if you have property abutting sidewalks or trails.
- **Organize a neighborhood cleanup day,** or just take a bag and pick up trash on your normal walking routes. Always clear your sidewalk of snow or debris.
- **Be a considerate driver.** Set an example: Drive at safe speeds in neighborhoods, let pedestrians cross at intersections, don't stop in crosswalks.
- **Notify the animal control officer of problem animals,** and the police of suspicious activity. Report street or signal lights that are out to the department of public works.

CHANGE YOUR COMMUNITY

- **Speak up at governance and planning meetings.** Demand bicycle- and pedestrian-friendly planning, engineering, and policies. For detailed information: Pedestrian and Bicycle Information Center, 877-WALK-BIKE; **www.pedbikeinfo.org**.
- National Center for Bicycling and Walking, 202-463-6622; **www.bikewalk.org**.
- The Robert Wood Johnson Foundation (RWJF) Active Living by Design Program: **www.activelivingbydesign.org**.
- America Walks, the national pedestrian advocacy organization: **www.americawalks.org**.

BUILD A TRAIL

- Learn how trails improve health: **www.cdc.gov/nccdphp/dnpa/physical/trails.htm**.
- Get a railroad right-of-way turned into a trail; contact the Rails-to-Trails Conservancy for assistance at 800-888-7747; 202-331-9696; **www.railtrails.org**.

GET KIDS WALKING TO SCHOOL

- Hold a Walk to School Day event; **www.walktoschool.org**.
- Set up a walking school bus, where adults walk with children daily. Request the CDC's *KidsWalk-to-School* booklet at 888-CDC-4NRG, or ccdinfo@cdc.gov.

BE A ROLE MODEL: WALK SOMEWHERE EVERY DAY

Encourage others by your actions. For a detailed resource list and comprehensive information on starting or maintaining a walking program, take a look at *The Complete Guide to Walking for Health, Weight Loss, and Fitness* by Mark Fenton (The Lyons Press, 2001).

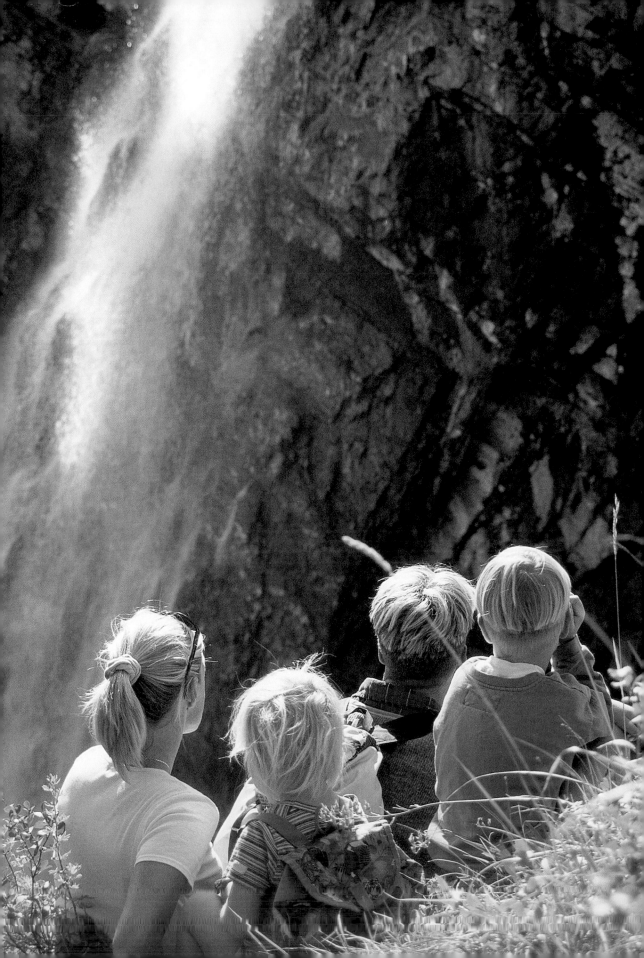

10 Reasons to Make a More Walkable World for You and Your Child

Just in case you have any doubt that it's worth your time, here are 10 quick reasons you and your child need a more walkable community (all based on research):

1. Health. You'll all be healthier if you walk more, and you'll walk more if there are better places to walk.

2. Economics. Local businesses do better when residents walk and shop locally, rather than driving to distant malls.

3. Housing values. Your home will be worth more in a safer, more walkable community (providing a better inheritance).

4. Safety. You'll be ready to walk day or night, and Grandma and Grandpa will be able to come visit and take the kids for a walk and you won't worry. Eventually you'll be able to let your children explore and develop with the freedom that earlier generations enjoyed.

5. Cleaner air. Car trips create a huge amount of air pollution, and childhood asthma rates are skyrocketing; the air quality around schools is especially at risk.

6. Cleaner water. The oil and fluids from cars run off the roads, and into the water in your communities. Fewer car trips means less soil and water pollution.

7. Less congestion. Every time someone walks, it means there's one less car on the road when you *do* have to drive; the road system works better when we walk and bike more.

8. Quieter streets. We've become accustomed to the roar of the automobile, instead of the ring of the bicycle bell or the shouts of street hockey; kids should be the sounds we hear in our neighborhoods, not engines and tires.

9. Less stress. Not every trip will require strapping into the car seat and white-knuckling it through stop lights.

10. Quality of life. Walk more and you and your children will know your neighbors, and they'll know you. See them often, and you'll look out for each other the way we all used to. And your children will feel like part of a community. Don't doubt that it's possible—we're lucky enough to live in such a place, and you should be, too.

TIP:

Use weekend walks for a change of scenery. Long weekend hikes clear the mind and burn calories.

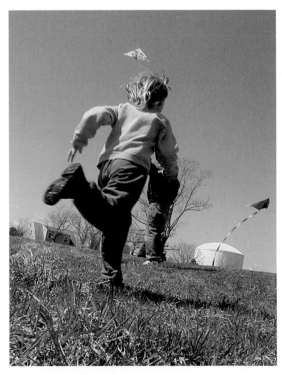

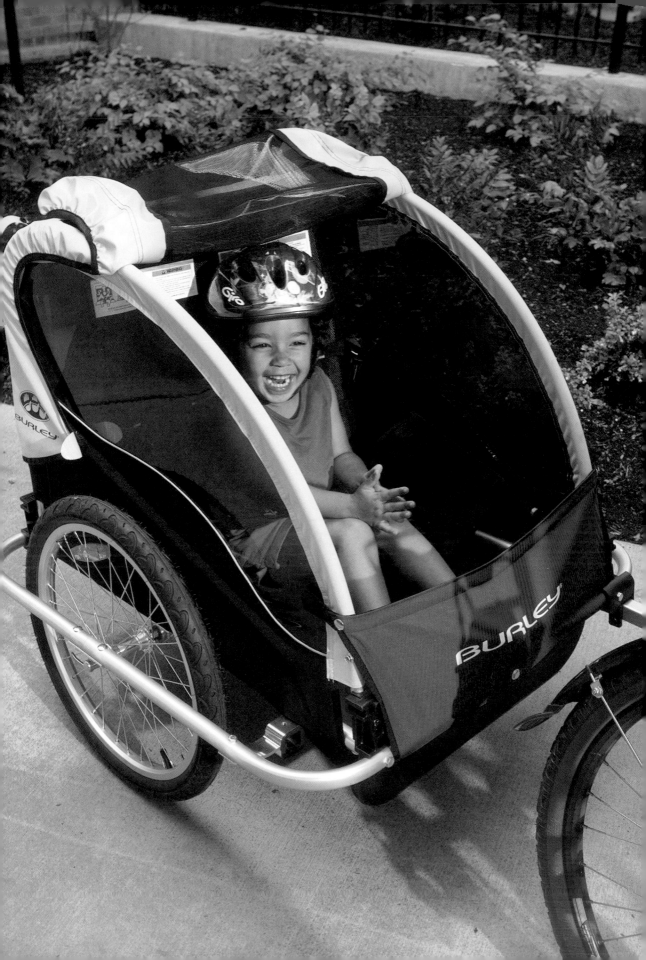

Gear 707:
Your Next Set of Wheels

Bike Seats and Trailers

Over the next months and years, you're going to want to expand your options beyond walking, hiking, and jogging. By adding bicycling to the mix, you can easily triple the distance you can cover in a given amount of time. Suddenly places you could never walk in 25 minutes are within reach, and you can leave the car behind (and get a dual-purpose workout) even more often.

There are fantastic carrier options that enable parents to cycle with their kids. Child seats, bicycle trailers, and tandem attachments are each aimed at children of different ages, so there's potential for several years of active riding together until your child can pedal on his own. But because of the potential for collision and falling is much greater when you add balance and traffic to the mix, it's essential to take a long look at safety when you choose your equipment. The safety considerations fall into three areas: the age of your child and her developmental readiness for the given carrier, your skills and experience and where you plan to ride, and the safety and sturdiness of the carrier you choose.

BICYCLE CHILD SEATS

These hard-shell plastic seats attach to a shelflike rack (sometimes included) that is in turn attached to the back of the adult bicycle at the frame and rear wheel. The padded seats are high on the sides and at the back for protection, and are equipped with a three- or five-point harness plus a padded lap bar, and molded footrests.

Your child is ready to ride in a bike seat when she can sit up on her own, has good body control (crawls, pulls up), and can support the weight of a bike helmet. Generally, this is all in place at about 12 months of age. Most seats are built to carry children up to 40 pounds.
Cost: $30–$180.
Upside: The child rides close to the parent for easy communication. Bike maneuvering is little changed by the seat.
Downside: The bike is not as stable with a seat and child. It can be difficult to get on and off your bike. The biggie: If you fall, your child falls, too.
Look for: A seat that meets ASTM standards. Simple in and out for child. Easy attach/detach if you plan to ride your bike without the seat sometimes. Generally, high-end seats have more padding and straps that are more adjustable and comfortable for the child. When you look at

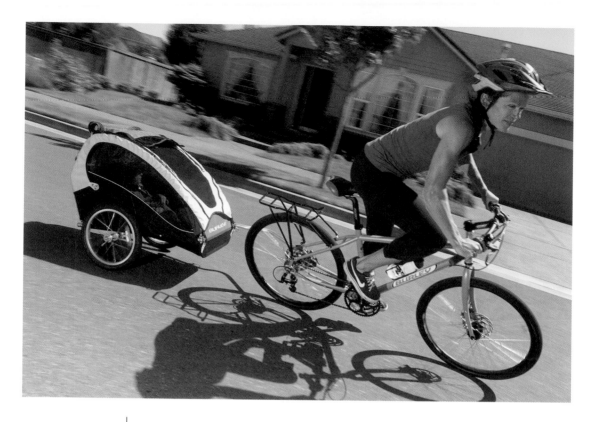

pricing, consider that buying a rear rack on which to mount the seat separately costs roughly $25–$60.

Nice extras: A seat that reclines slightly and that has a rest or notch to accommodate the child's helmet is a plus. A new feature—suspension—adds comfort over potholes, railroad tracks, and curbs.

Brands include: Co-Pilot, Bell, Kettler, Rhode Gear, Topeak.

BICYCLE TRAILERS

Bicycle trailers let you tow one or two children behind a full-sized adult bike. The enclosed pod hitches to the parent's bike via a long arm, and sits on two bicycle-style wheels. Some are full plastic shells, others are more of a lighweight frame with cross pieces and webbing. All have a plastic and fabric canopy; some come with various screen and window combinations.

Most trailers come with or have the option to buy a converter that lets you transform the trailer to a three-wheeled stroller. Trailers tend to be their best as such, but conversions can be convenient for getting around on foot once you've biked to your destination. They're probably the best choice if you'll primarily use them for cycling, and will convert the trailer to a stroller occasionally. If you do plan on walking a lot with a converted bike trailer, try it out that way first to make sure that the weight or a wobbly front wheel doesn't drive you nutty.

Most bike trailers are loaded with safety features and designed for use on the road, including a tall flag and lots of reflective material. But your bike will have a 5-foot (or more) extension behind it and will turn and stop differently, so it's best

✳TIP:

Walk a mile in 20 minutes and burn about 90 calories. Walk 2 miles in 30 minutes and burn about 200 calories. Walk 5 miles in an hour and burn up to 500 calories.

to first use a trailer on bike paths, rail-trails, and other places where you'll meet few cars, at least until you really get the hang of your new ride.

Children need to be independent sitters as well as show body control by pulling up and crawling before they're candidates for bike trailers. Most hit the mark by 12 months.

Cost: $150–$450.

Upside: Because they're low to the ground and don't affect the bike's stability, trailers don't pose the risk of a fall. They can carry two, whereas a bike seat is built for one.

Downside: May tip over, particularly when turning sharply. Though trailers are brightly colored and bear safety flags, cars may have trouble spotting them. They're bulky, and so may be hard to provide safe clearance for other traffic and obstacles. Towing a trailer and passenger is hard work, especially uphill, and the brake response time is slower.

Look for: ASTM safety approval. Complete roll cage made of strong, rigid materials, such as aluminum or steel. A zippered canopy that offers sun, weather, and splatter protection. High sides or wheel guards so a sleeping child won't press the side of the trailer into the wheels. A flexible hitch that keeps the trailer upright even if your bike hits the ground, and that includes a backup attachment in case trailer and bike part ways. A comfortable, adjustable five-point safety harness. Adequate and adjustable ventilation; comfortable, roomy seats. A warranty. Aluminum wheels (they're lighter and track better than polymer). If you want to use your trailer for both walking and cycling, look for a model with a convenient conversion and a large front wheel (at least 12 inches in diameter) that sits close to the trailer, not far out in front. The front wheel should be fixed, not swiveling, to avoid a wobbly ride.

Nice extras: A panel or notch that accommodates the child's helmet comfortably (you can also find flat-back helmets in lieu of this). Reclining seats. Large windows. Storage compartment for toys, snacks, extra clothing. A model that's easy to fold and set up—especially if you'll be storing or traveling with the trailer.

Brands include: Bell, Burley, Chariot Carriers, Kool-Stop, InSTEP, Schwinn, Trek, Wike.

YOUR CHILD'S FIRST RIDE

Given that getting into a bike trailer will be an unfamiliar experience, you want to be extra sensitive to how your child is feeling on the first few rides. Here are tips for loading up the first few times, from John Kluge, sales manager at Burley, a trailer manufacturer. The trick with young children on the first few outings is have as much as possible ready to roll *before* putting your child's bike helmet on.

1. First connect the trailer to the bike.

TIP:
Scramble up rocks to improve your agility. Walk in sand or shallow water to boost calorie burn. Tightrope-walk the lines of a track occasionally, for balance.

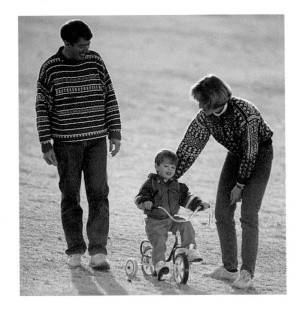

2. Then stow any toys or supplies (diaper bag, food).
3. Add the child and connect the harness system.
4. Finally, put on the child's helmet. Be extra careful not to catch a pudgy little cheek in the clasp (it's easy to do—put your finger between the clip and her skin), or you'll struggle to get it on next time.
5. Take off right away. "Most small children don't really like the helmet, so if you can get it on and then quickly distract them with the motion of the trailer it usually works out," John suggests. "Later they'll associate using the helmet with something fun, and it won't be a problem."

Take It from Us:

Always do the ABC–Quick Check before getting on a bike. *Always!*

"A recent over-the-handlebars crash after a family bike ride (fortunately my daughter, Skye, was not on the trailer bike at the time) reminded me that I should never take anything for granted when bicycling. No car was involved; my brakes just failed. But I was horrified to think what might have happened if I did have Skye along. As a result, we never start a bike ride—even just down the street to a friend's—without doing the following one-minute safety check.

"Do the ABC–Quick Check before every bike ride:

- *A—Air.* Make sure tires are fully inflated with a quick thumb squeeze.
- *B—Brakes.* Give both brakes a hard squeeze, push the bike forward and back, and make sure they're grabbing the tires with full force. (This would have saved me a lot of grief.)
- *C—Crank.* Check that the crank arms (the things the pedals are attached to), pedals, and chain are all in good shape and nothing's loose.
- *Quick Check.* Most bikes have quick-release bolts on the front tire and seat post; some, on brake cables and other spots. Check that all quick releases are firmly set and no parts are loose.

"Trust me—it's worth the 90 seconds it takes to do this every time you hop aboard.

—*Mark*

TRAILER BIKES

These clever creatures allow kids as young as four to pedal right behind Mom or Dad on what looks like a bike and a half. The child rides on a bike with his own pedals, rear wheel, and fixed handlebars—but no front wheel. The unit attaches to the adult bike's seat post or a special rear rack (included), and the passenger can choose to pedal or not. There are geared and nongeared versions. Depending on your child's independence and strength, he may want to pedal his own bike between ages five and seven, but some use trailer bikes until age 10 (depending on the unit's weight limit).

Cost: $250–$350.

Upside: Allows parent and child to ride farther together. Helps the child build balance, increase strength, and learn cycling skills and how to deal with traffic.

Downside: Can't be used unless attached to adult bike, and if you fall, so does your passenger. Adds work and changes maneuvering (slightly wider turns and longer stopping distance) for the adult.

Look for: An easy-to-attach, strong, secure hitch with a device to slow the fall of the child's bike in the event that your bike falls or tips.

Nice extras: Gears that help older children learn and practice shifting.

Brands include: Adams, B.O.B., Burley, InSTEP, Kiddopotamus, Schwinn, Trek, Xtracycle, Yakima.

PLAY IT SAFE: SAFETY TIPS FOR BIKE TRAILERS AND SEATS

The Basics

▪ Read and follow the manufacturer's directions. Knowing your gear inside and out is the first step toward keeping your little passenger safe.

▪ Check and follow the manufacturer's age and weight recommendations.

▪ Leave ample time to set up before a ride. That way, you won't miss an important step or strap because you're rushing.

▪ Before each outing, check the trailer and hitch or seat and your bike to make sure there is no damage. Make sure the brakes are working properly and the tires have adequate air pressure.

▪ Dress your child for the weather, keeping in mind that because she's sitting still, she won't warm up as you ride like you will.

▪ Make sure your child has a properly fitting helmet and that he wears it every time he's in the trailer, no exceptions. Set a good example by wearing one yourself.

▪ Make sure the child's harness is attached securely and adjusted properly before each outing.

▪ Hitch the trailer before you put your child in.

▪ Clean up. Scrub it out about twice a year with a bucket of warm water, a biodegradable soap (Simple Green), and a soft brush. Hose it out and make sure it dries before putting it away in a dark place like the garage.

With Baby on Board

▪ When you ride with baby in a bike seat, remember that it will be tougher to balance with the extra weight behind you. Compensate for this by getting on and off with caution, and starting and stopping slowly and carefully.

▪ Regularly check on your passenger to make sure her position is safe and that she's comfortable.

▪ Be vigilant anytime you're riding in or near traffic and follow the rules of the road. Assume that drivers *don't* see you.

▪ Remember that a trailer adds length to your bike, and you'll need to allow extra time for street

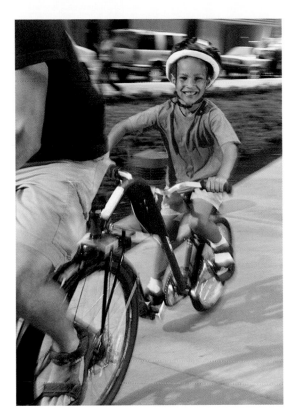

crossings, slightly wider turns, and so on.

▪ Allow extra time for braking with a trailer, particularly in wet conditions.

▪ Don't leave your child in a trailer without supervision.

▪ Don't set or strap an infant car seat into a bike trailer or child bicycle seat.

▪ Keep the ride smooth for younger children by sticking to smooth roads and surfaces.

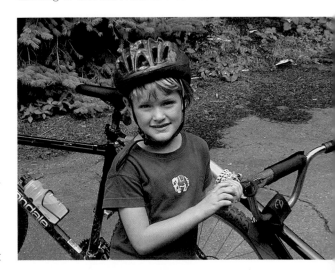

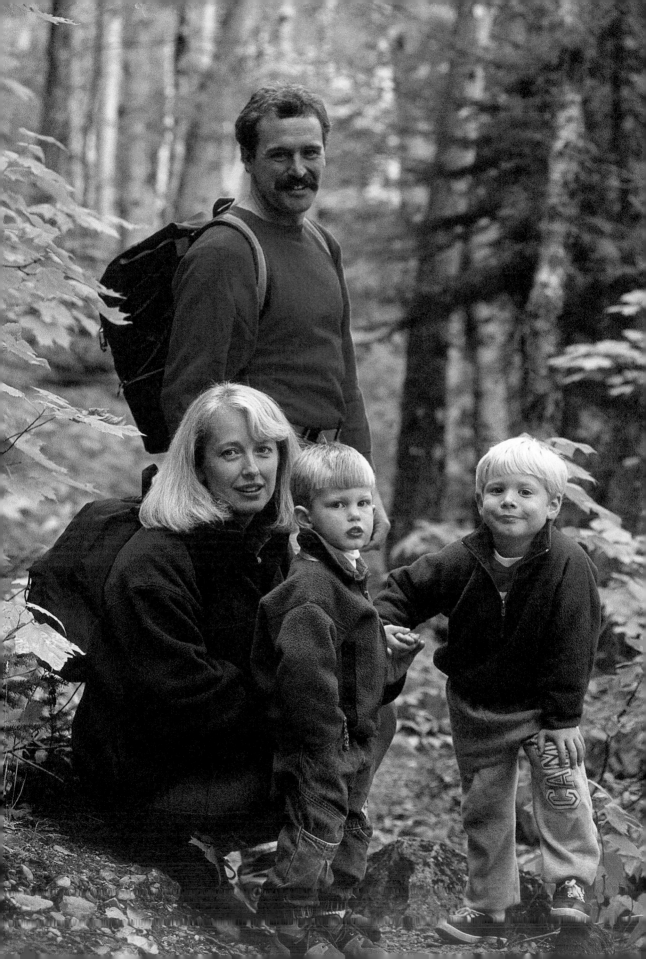

Walking as a Way of Life

21

It's What You Were (Both) Born For

Here it is, the final installment in our recommended walking program. But it's anything but the end—it's really the beginning of a new active lifestyle. New because even if you were active before pregnancy, you're now doing it with a new member in your family. And we can boil down all the advice, exercise minutes, stretches, and strength moves into a single point: Walking is what your body is made for. You should be doing it every day, as much as you can, however you can, whenever you can. Some is good and more is better. Longer will help make you trim; faster will help firm your muscles and strengthen your heart. And doing it every single day will do the most important thing: establish to your child that it should be integral to his life, too. One of the best things you can do for yourself, and one of the finest gifts you can give your youngster, is walking.

The Walking Pyramid has shown you all the physical activity recommendations for health, weight loss, and fitness in fairly standard exercise form: *so many minutes at such-and-such an intensity*, or *so many steps on the pedometer*. But this version of the pyramid is laid out to remind you how you can live a life laced with walking, and still meet all the "exercise" criteria.

GENERAL REMINDERS FOR POSTMESTER IV AND BEYOND

You know it all already, but here it is one last time:

- Walk every day, at least 30 minutes. Break it up if you want, but be sure that the bare minimum happens daily.
- Stretch—even just a few minutes—after as many walks as possible.
- When you have time, walk longer. Target 45 to 60 minutes (more if you can) a few days of the week.
- Do some sort of resistance training to keep muscles toned and strong, and your posture tall and healthy.
- Walk faster, especially when time is tight. Speed is the great equalizer; use it to cover more distance so walking is viable for errands, and to turn a short walk into a workout.
- Seek variety. Do all the other stuff you like: bike, swim, play tennis or soccer, take aerobics, Spin. But don't stop walking.

The Walking Pyramid

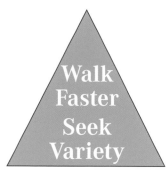

Walk Faster Seek Variety

GOAL: FITNESS

WHAT YOU MIGHT DO: 2 DAYS TAKE A FAST 20-MIN. WALK TO STORE, BANK.
PLAY TENNIS 2–4 TIMES/MONTH; BIKE OFTEN FOR ERRANDS.

Walk Longer Build Strength

GOAL: WEIGHT LOSS

WHAT YOU MIGHT DO: ONE LONG WALK WITH STROLLER; PLUS WEEKEND FAMILY HIKE.
3 DAYS GO TO GYM, OR LIFT WEIGHTS AT HOME.

Walk Daily Stretch Often

GOAL: HEALTH

WHAT YOU MIGHT DO: 3 DAYS WALK KIDS TO AND FROM SCHOOL.
QUICK STRETCH MOST DAYS; FULL STRETCH TWICE A WEEK.

WEEKLY GOALS FOR THE LOW-KEY PROGRAM

▪ Do the sample week and you'll manage 200 minutes of exercise this week—well beyond the surgeon general's minimum recommendation for long-term health.

▪ At least once a week, try for a walk of 45 minutes or longer .

▪ Try for some speed on three of your shorter walks. Go easy for the first 5 minutes, speed up for the middle 15 to 20 minutes, then cool down for the last 5 minutes. Target a brisk pace: 3.5 to 4.0 mph or faster, or an RPE of 5 to 7.

▪ Keep stretching often—the quick stretches when time is short, the full stretches if you feel you need more.

▪ Build strength. Do the full strength routine twice a week, and the core routine on two other days.

A TYPICAL WEEK NEAR THE END OF POSTMESTER IV, LOW-KEY PROGRAM:							
	MON.	TUES.	WED.	THUR.	FRI.	SAT.	SUN.
WALK (minutes)	30 (B)	40	30 (B)	35	20 (B)	45+	OFF
OTHER STUFF	CORE	FULL STRENGTH		CORE	FULL STRENGTH		

"B" is a brisk walk, 3.5–4.0 mph or more.

low-key program

MODERATE PROGRAM, POSTMESTER IV

WEEKLY GOALS FOR THE MODERATE PROGRAM

- The sample week gives a total of about 250 minutes of walking a week—an average of more than 40 minutes for six days of walking.

- At least two days a week, shoot for at least 45 minutes of walking, even if it's broken up. On a third day, go for a 60-minute walk or more.

- Walk for speed on three of your shorter walks. Go easy for the first 5 minutes, speed up for the middle 20 to 25 minutes, then cool down for the last 5 minutes. For two of those, target a brisk pace (RPE of 5 to 7); on the third, go for a fast tempo (RPE of 7 to 9).

- Do the quick stretches after every walk; when you feel you need it, make it the full stretch routine.

- Get stronger. Do the full strength routine three times a week, and the short core strength routine one or two other days.

A TYPICAL WEEK NEAR THE END OF POSTMESTER IV, MODERATE PROGRAM:							
	MON.	TUES.	WED.	THUR.	FRI.	SAT.	SUN.
WALK (minutes)	35 (B)	50	25 (F)	45	35 (B)	60+	OFF
OTHER STUFF	FULL STRENGTH	CORE	FULL STRENGTH	CORE	FULL STRENGTH		

"B" is a brisk walk, 3.5-4.0 mph or more; "F" is fast, better than 4.0 mph at the least.

CHALLENGING PROGRAM, POSTMESTER IV

WEEKLY GOALS FOR THE CHALLENGING PROGRAM

▪ Do the sample week and you'll collect an impressive 300 minutes of walking. That's the equivalent of walking an hour on five days of the week, and that's not counting any time you devote to stretching and strengthening. This is nothing less than a full-fledged, athletic fitness program. Don't panic—some of your walking can be woven into trips for errands, to see friends, and so on. Plus, much of it can be piled into a few longer walks each week.

▪ Mix your walking up; don't feel stuck at 75 minutes on the weekend, just because that's what is written. If you have the time and spirit for it, take your baby for a two-hour hike and picnic.

▪ When time is tight, walk fast. On three days a week, go for speed; on one, target a brisk pace (5 to 7 RPE), but on two go for blazing speed (7 to 9 RPE). Begin and end with 5 minutes of easy walking, but in the middle let it rip.

▪ Keep stretching daily. Do the quick stretches often, the full stretches whenever you're inclined.

▪ Stay strong. Continue resistance training at least three days a week; add more if you vary your routines from day to day (say, upper-body exercises on one day, lower-body the next).

A TYPICAL WEEK NEAR THE END OF POSTMESTER IV, CHALLENGING PROGRAM:							
	MON.	**TUES.**	**WED.**	**THUR.**	**FRI.**	**SAT.**	**SUN.**
WALK (minutes)	30 (F)	60	45 (F)	60	30 (B)	75+	OFF
OTHER STUFF	FULL STRENGTH	CORE	FULL STRENGTH	CORE	FULL STRENGTH	CORE	

"B" is a brisk walk, 3.5–4.0 mph or more; "F" is fast, better than 4.0 mph at the least.

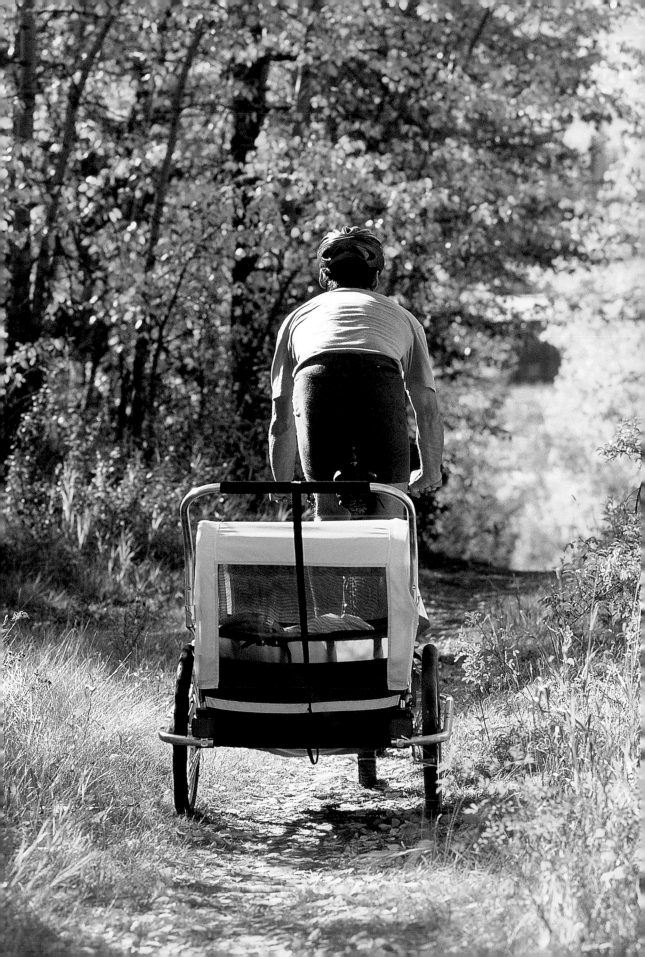

Take It from Us:

You can stay active even while writing a book together!

Yeah, we thought it would be fun, too. But check out this schedule in the Fenton house at the peak of writing intensity—the weeks before deadline. We had three goals: (1) Keep everybody active and healthy, including son Max (8, in second grade) and daughter Skye (5, in half-day kindergarten). (2) Write a great book. (3) Not kill each other.

"We're proud of our success on number 1 and hope you like number 2. Frankly, Mark's a little worried about the third one. Anyway, here's a typical day in the lives, trying to practice what we preach:

"7:30 A.M. Everybody up. One parent gets everyone breakfast, dressed; the other hits the computer.

"8:30 A.M. Mark out the door with Max for 10-minute bike ride to school; then ride to town hall to sign documents (Mark's on the planning board, trying to do all the wacky 'walkable community' stuff), then bank, and home.

"9:30 A.M. Lisa updates Mark on writing; dashes out for 45-minute workout at the gym; Mark on computer (Shower? Nah!). Skye plays with a friend.

"10:30 A.M. Lisa back. Each on a computer researching, writing, editing, with interruptions from kids ('Can we have a snack?'), telephone ('We'd like to confirm a speaking engagement . . .'), and each other ('Where'd you put the stuff on walking shoes?' 'Me? You had it last').

"10:47 A.M. Disagree over layout of a section of chapter 13. Nursing vs. exercise physiology. Lisa wins.

"Noon. Brief lunch break with Skye.

"12:17 P.M. Heated discussion re: placement of 'real mom' advice boxes. Lisa wins.

"12:30 P.M. Lisa out the door to school with Skye on trailer bike. On the way home swings by store for printer cartridge (going through them like popcorn).

"1:15 P.M. Back to dueling computers.

"2:07 P.M. Argue over section titles. Lisa wins. (See a theme here?)

"3:00 P.M. Mark off on trailer bike to pick up kids. All ride to store, get groceries for supper.

"3:45 P.M. Back to computers ('What do you mean you can't format a table?'); kids play.

"5:00 P.M. Lisa bangs out supper; eat together.

"6:00 P.M. Dishes piled; Max homework, Skye play, Lisa and Mark work.

"7:30 P.M. Bedtime routine with kids.

"8:30 P.M. Back to dueling computers until whenever.

"Despite the zaniness, everyone got in some exercise and ate decent meals. In fact, exercise may have been the key safety valve that kept things running smoothly.

"One final thought: Thank God Tracy did all the hard work. She's our hero.

— Mark and Lisa

Resources

Reading List

Here are some of the books related to pregnancy, postpartum life, and active living in general that we've found most useful as parents, or that we used as references in this work. It is by no means a complete list, but it is a good starting point if you've just learned you're pregnant.

Anderson, Bob. *Stretching*. Bolinas, Calif.: Shelter Publications, 1980. Easy to use, very simple with clear illustrations, still considered by many a definitive handbook on static stretching for just about any activity.

Eisenberg, Arlene, Heidi E. Murkoff, and Sandee E. Hathaway. *What to Expect When You're Expecting*. New York: Workman Publishing Co., 1991. A classic standby for expectant moms, full of answers to every pregnancy question you'd think to ask.

Fenton, Mark. *The Complete Guide to Walking for Health, Weight Loss, and Fitness*. Guilford, Conn.: Lyons Press, 2001. Okay, tooting our own horn here, but this goes into lots of detail on walking for exercise; specific workout recommendations; a detailed one-year, day-by-day exercise program; cross-training activities; hiking and racewalking; and injury prevention and treatment. It also has a one-year training log woven into the book.

Ferber, Richard, M.D. S*olve Your Child's Sleep Problems*. New York: Simon and Schuster, 1985. The author is the director of the Center for Pediatric Sleep Disorders at the Children's Hospital in Boston. The bible on getting your kids, and, therefore, you, onto a regular schedule.

Kunstler, James H. *Home from Nowhere*. New York: Simon and Schuster, 1996. Neither a pregnancy nor fitness book, this is an enjoyable and readable treatise on the need to build more "walkability" into our communities. Kunstler is highly opinionated, but it's an opinion that anyone who cares about his or her child's health and welfare should take seriously.

Miller, Olivia H. *The Prenatal Yoga Deck*. San Francisco: Chronicle Books, 2003. Fifty cards show you pregnancy appropriate yoga moves; coded by trimester. (800) 722-6657; www.chroniclebooks.com.

Ross, Cindy, and Todd Gladfelter. *Kids in the Wild: A Family Guide to Outdoor Recreation*. Seattle: The Mountaineers Books, 1995. Great insights into successfully introducing children to the outdoors.

Pregnancy and Baby-Related Information and Gear

This is a quick summary of many of the places you can turn to for more information on pregnancy and baby-related gear.

MATERNITY AND POSTDELIVERY WORKOUT APPAREL

Athleta. For sports bras only. 888-322-5515; www.athleta.com

Babystyle. Sells the Belly Basics line. 877-378-9537; www.babystyle.com

Fit Maternity. 888-961-9100; www.fitmaternity.com

Hind. Athletic gear for women; not maternity wear, but great sports bra offerings. 800-952-4463; www.hind.com

Liz Lange for Nike. 888-616-5757; www.lizlange.com

Mothers in Motion. Much of the maternity apparel pictured in the book is from M.I.M. 877-512-8800; www.mothers-in-motion.com

The Power of Two, by adidas. 866-679-0143; www.ThePowerofTwo.net

Reebok. 866-271-5859; www.reebok.com

Title 9. 800-342-4448; www.title9sports.com

CARRIERS

Both soft-front carriers and hard-frame backpack carriers, as noted.

Baby Björn (soft carriers). 800-593-5522; www.regallager

Evenflo (both styles). 800-233-5921; www.evenflo.com

Kelty (both styles). 800-423-2320; www.kelty.com

Maclaren (soft carriers). 877-442-4622; www.maclarenbaby.com

REI. 800-426-4840; www.rei.com

Tough Traveler (backpack carriers). 800-go-tough; www.toughtraveler.com

STRENGTH AND STRETCHING GEAR

Ball Dynamics International, Inc. 800-752-2255; www.balldynamics.com

Megafitness. 800-925-2772; www.megafitness.com

OPTP. 888-819-0121; www.optp.com

Perform Better. 888-556-7464, www.performbetter.com

Reebok. 866-271-5859, www.reebokdirect.com

SPRI Products, Inc. 800-222-7774, www.spriproducts.com

BIKE-RELATED GEAR

Adams (Trail a Bike). www.norco.com/adams

Bell (helmets, child seats). 800-456-2355; www.bellsports.com

Burley (trailers, trailer bikes). 866-248-5634; www.burley.com

Chariot Carriers (trailers). 800-262-8651; www.chariotcarriers.com

InSTEP (trailers). 800-242 6110; www.instep.net

Kettler (child seats). 757-427 2400; www.kettlerusa.com

Kool-Stop (trailers). 800-586-3332; www.koolstop.com

REI (carries all gear). 800-426-4840; www.rei.com

Rhode Gear (child seats). 888-266-3085; www.rhodegear.com

Schwinn (trailers). 800-242-6110; www.instep.net

Todson, for Topeak (child seats). 800-213-4561; www.topeak.com

Trek (trailers). 920-478-4678; www.trekbikes.com

Wike (trailers). 866-584-9452; wicycle.com

STROLLERS

Aprica. 310-639-6387; www.apricausa.com

Bertini. 800-SIMO-4-ME; www.bertinistrollers.com

Britax. 888-427-4829; www.britaxusa.com

Bugaboo. 800-460-2922; www.bugaboo.nl/us

Chicco. 877-424-4226; www.chiccousa.com

Combi. 800-992-6624; www.combi-intl.com

Cosco. 800-314-9327; www.coscoinc.com

Dorel Juvenile Group (Eddie Bauer, Safety 1st). 800-544-1108; www.djgusa.com

Emmaljunga. www.emmaljung.no

Evenflo. 800-233-5921; www.evenflo.com

Fisher Price. 800-432-5437; www.fisher-price.com

Graco. 800-345-4109; www.gracobaby.com

Inglesina. 877-486-5112; www.inglesina.com

Kolcraft. 800-453-7673; www.kolcraft.com

Maclaren. 877-442-4622; www.maclarenbaby.com

Mountain Buggy (distributed by Sycamore Kids). 866-524-8805; www.mountainbuggyusa.com

Peg Perego. 800-671-1701; www.perego.com

Safety 1st (Dorel Juvenile Group). 800-909-7133; www.safety1st.com

Schwinn by InSTEP. 800-242-6110; www.instep.net

Silver Cross. 866-887-9642; www.silvercrossbaby.com

Zooper (Grand Enterprises). 888-742-9899; www.zooper.com

JOGGING STROLLERS

Baby Jogger. 800-241-1848; www.babyjogger.com

Baby Trend. 800-328-7363; www.babytrend.com

BOB Stroller. 800-893-2447; www.bobgear.com

Dreamer Design. 800-278-9626; www.dreamerdesign.net

InSTEP. 800-242-6110; www.instep.net

Kelty. 800-423-2320; www.kelty.com

Kool Stride. 800-586-3332; www.koolstop.com

Schwinn (by InSTEP). 800-242-6110; www.instep.net

MISCELLANEOUS OTHER

CamelBak Products, Inc. 800-767-8725; www.camelbak.com

Mobile Moms (for the Toastie Toddler, a liner/zip-around sack for your stroller/jogger). 212-685-0935; www.mobilemoms.com

Stroller Strides (classes for moms and babies). 800-FIT-4MOM; www.strollerstrides.com

General Walking and Fitness-Related Information and Gear

Here are some more broad resources to support your lifelong walking habit.

EVENTS, CLUBS, AND WALKING ORGANIZATIONS

American Diabetes Association's Team Diabetes Walks. Walk or run a marathon (26.2 miles). Minimum donation is $3,000 to $4,000, depending on your choice of location: Chicago, Disney World, Dublin, Las Vegas, Kona, Maui, San Francisco, Rome, Quebec, Ottawa, and Vancouver. Call 888-342-2383 or visit www.diabetes.org/teamdiabetes.

American Heart Association (AHA). American Heart Walk is the AHA's premiere walking and fund-raising event that takes place in more than 1,000 cities every year. The event focuses on preventing heart disease and stroke by raising money to support research and heart-healthy lifestyle programs. This noncompetitive event typically occurs on the last weekend of September or first weekend of October. Call 800-AHA-USA1 (800-242-8721) or visit www.american heart.org/health/lifestyle/american_heart_walk/benefits.html.

American Volksport Association (AVA). AVA's 500 clubs organize more than 3,000 events per year nationwide. To find a club or event near you, call 800-830-WALK (800-830-9255) or visit www.ava.org.

Arthritis Foundation's Joints in Motion Event. Walk or run a marathon (26.2 miles). Airfare, hotels, and entry fees are covered if you meet your fund-raising goal. Minimum pledges range from $2,500 to $5,000, depending on your choice of location: New Orleans, Vancouver, Dublin, and Honolulu. Call 800-960-7682 or visit www.arthritis.org.

Avon's 3-Day Breast Cancer Walks. Sixty-mile group walks including food, tent accommodations, and entertainment. Minimum pledge is $1,800. Event locations: Atlanta, Boston, Chicago, Los Angeles, New York, San Francisco, and Washington, D.C. Call 888-332-9286 or visit www.avoncrusade.com.

Leukemia Society of America Marathons. Walk or run a marathon (26.2 miles). Airfare, hotels, and entry fees are covered if you meet your fund-raising goal. Minimum pledge varies with event; there are more than 30 events in this series. Call 800-482-TEAM (800-482-8326) or visit www.lsa-team intraining.org.

March of Dimes WalkAmerica. The March of Dimes' biggest fund-raiser, WalkAmerica supports lifesaving research and community programs that save babies from birth defects, low birth weight, and infant death. WalkAmerica will take place in 1,400 communities in all 50 states, the District of Columbia, and Puerto Rico. In most communities WalkAmerica is held at the end of April. Routes vary in length, but most are about 20 kilometers (approximately 12 miles). Call 800-525-WALK (800-525-9255) from January through April, call the national MOD office at 914-428-7100 any time during the year, or visit www.modimes.org.

MS Walk. The MS Walk will be offered in 700 cities across the nation, with distances from 3 to 12 miles; accessible routes are always available. Complimentary food, beverages, first aid, and special transportation provided. Call 800-FIGHT-MS (800-344-4867) or visit www.nmss.org.

Race for the Cure. The Komen Race for the Cure series has become the largest series of 5K and 1-mile run/fitness walks in the nation. It was held in 108 cities across the country in 2000, with more than one million participants expected. Proceeds fund both national research efforts and local breast cancer initiatives. Call 888-603-RACE (888-603-7223) or visit www.raceforthecure.com.

FOOTWEAR

Athletic Footwear

Most of the companies below have online catalogs and store-finder features on their Web sites.

Adidas. 800-448-1796; www.adidas.com

Asics. 800-678-9435; www.asicstiger.com

Avia. 888-855-AVIA (888-855-2842); www.aviashoes.com

Easy Spirit. 800-EASY-242 (800-327-9242); no Web site available

New Balance. 800-253-SHOE (800-253-7463); www.newbalance.com

Nike. 800-344-6453; www.nike.com

Puma. 800-662-PUMA (800-662-7862); www.puma.com

Reebok. 800-843-4444; www.reebok.com

Ryka. 888-834-RYKA (888-834-7952); www.ryka.com

Saucony. 800-365-7282; www.saucony.com

Teva. 800-FOR-TEVA (800-367-8382); www.teva.com

Rugged Footwear

These shoes and boots are more suited to the trail; also see hiking outfitters below.

Hi-Tec. 800-521-1698; www.hi-tec.com

L.L.Bean. 800-221-4221; www.llbean.com

Merrell. 888-637-7001; www.merrellboot.com

Montrail. 800-647-0224; www.montrail.com

Rockport. 888-ROCKPORT (888-762-5767); www.rockport.com

Tecnica. 800-258-3897; www.tecnicausa.com

Timberland. 800-445-5545; www.timberland.com

Vasque. 800-224-HIKE (800-224-4453); www.vasque.com

Heart Rate Monitors

Acumen. Acumen Basix Plus model monitors heart rate and even calculates your target range. 800-852-7823; www.acumeninc.com

Creative Health Products. Discounted health products; free information, catalog, and pricing when you call. 800-742-4478; www.chponline.com

CardioSport. All monitors are water resistant to 20 meters and have handlebar adapters for use on indoor fitness equipment. 888-760-3059; www.cardiosport.com

Polar. Waterproof and long battery life; personal trainer, coaching tips, and special-events sections on its Web page. 800-227-1314; www.polarusa.com

HIKING—CONTACTS, INFORMATION, AND OUTDOOR OUTFITTERS

Hiking Organizations

American Hiking Society. A national hiking and trail advocacy organization that can help you get in touch with a club in your area. Call 301-565-6704 or visit www.americanhiking.org.

Appalachian Mountain Club. America's oldest conservation and recreation organization based in the northeastern United States. The AMC teaches skills, operates lodges, fixes trails, publishes guides, and works on conservation issues. To join a local chapter or get more information, call 617-523-0636 or visit www.outdoors.org.

Sierra Club. This well-known environmental organization provides information on current environmental issues, teaches conservation skills, and sponsors 330 national

and international outings per year. For more information, call the national office at 415-977-5500 or visit www.sierraclub.org.

Trail organizations

American Discovery Trail Society (Delaware to California). 800-663-2387; www.discoverytrail.org

Appalachian Trail Conference (East Coast). 304-535-6331; www.appalachiantrail.org

Continental Divide Trail Alliance (Rocky Mountain States). 888-909-CDTA (888-909-2382); www.cdtrail.org

The East Coast Greenway (from Florida to Maine). 401-789-4625; www.greenway.org/greenway.htm

North Country Trail Association (Great Lakes and upper Midwest). 616-454-5506; www.northcountry trail.org

Pacific Crest Trail Association. 888-PCTRAIL (888-728-7245); www.pcta.org

OUTDOOR OUTFITTERS AND OTHER GREAT RESOURCES

Mail-order catalogs

L.L.Bean: Call 800-441-5713 to request a catalog or visit www.llbean.com for clothing and gear, plus an international park-search feature.

REI: Call 800-426-4840 to request a catalog or visit www.rei.com for the gear shop, a learn and share feature, classes and events, and a link to the REI outlet store.

Web sites

www.altrec.com. Plenty of gear offerings, plus a how-to-buy feature. Links to other sports, such as cycling, climbing, paddling, and

snow sports. Live online service or call 800-369-3949.

www.backpacking.about.com. A wealth of information on outdoor gear, services, clubs, and organizations, plus links to related sites.

www.backroads.com. To plan an outdoors vacation, visit the Web site or call 800-GO-ACTIVE (800-462-2848).

www.4hiking.com. Gear, tips, trails and tours, and links to related sites, such as hiking and trail organizations.

www.greatoutdoors.com. Gear, weather, recipes, and tips for a variety of outdoor sports.

www.gorp.com. Plan a trip, buy gear and maps, read tips and articles about outdoor activities, find or rate a trail, or post a message on the discussion boards.

www.kidssource.com. This Web site caters to active outdoor families, providing information and gear for parents and children and helpful links to related sites.

www.outfittermag.com. Online version of the magazine. Check the outdoor directory for extensive listings of packs and bags, accessories, apparel, resources/media, and equipment.

www.planetoutdoors.com. Wide selection of gear, plus tips and articles.

PEDOMETERS

Accusplit. 800-935-1996; www.accusplit.com

NEW Lifestyles. 888-SIT-LESS (888-748-5377) or 816-353-1852; www.digiwalker.com

Optimal Health Products. 888-339-2067; www.intohealth.com

WALKING POLES

Exel. www.nordicwalking.com

Exerstrider. 800-554-0989; www.exerstrider.com

Leki. 800-255-9982; www.leki.com

RACEWALKING

North American Racewalking Foundation. NARF can provide people with racewalking tips and the names of coaches and contacts around the country. You can contact Elaine Ward, the group's managing director, at 626-441-5459 for referrals and educational materials, or visit the foundation's Web site at www.members.aol.com/rwnarf.

USA Track and Field. The national governing body for track and field and racewalking in the United States. To find your regional track and field office, which can connect you with your local racewalking chairperson and contacts for local walking clubs, contact the national office at USA Track and Field, P.O. Box 120, Indianapolis, Indiana 46206; 317-261-0500; www.race-walk.com.

SOCKS

One of the most mundane pieces of gear, yet one of the most important to a walker. You'll never regret making the investment in quality socks. Here are some brands I've found comfortable and durable over the years, but there are many others, as well.

Bridgedale. Sports-specific, durable socks for rugged activities. 888-797-6257; www.bridgedale-socks.co.uk

Fox River. Athletic, outdoor, and winter socks and liners. 800-247-1815; www.foxrivermills.com

Smart Wool. Made of natural wool fibers; socks and liners are available in sports-specific, outdoor, and casual styles. 800-550-WOOL (800-550-9665); www.smartwool.com

Thor•Lo. Sports-specific, outdoor, or casual socks. 888-THORLOS (888-846-7567); www.thorlo.com

TREADMILLS

This is an incomplete list, but it will get you started comparing some of the best hardware.

Cybex. 888-GO-CYBEX; www.ecybex.com

PaceMaster. 973-276-9700; www.pacemaster.com

Precor. 800-4-PRECOR (800-477-3267); www.precor.com

Schwinn. 800-SCHWINN; www.schwinn.com

True. 800-426-6570; www.truefitness.com

WALK TO SCHOOL DAY

This is usually the first Wednesday of October; get current information at www.walktoschool.org.

KidsWalk-to-School. A guide to promote walking to school, from the Centers for Disease Control. 888-CDC-4NRG; request by e-mail at ccdinfo@cdc.gov or download at www.cdc.gov/nccdphp/dnpa/kidswalk.htm. This information-packed booklet is designed for parents, educators, and community leaders hoping to organize children and adults to regularly and safely walk to school together. It offers a step-by-step approach for creating a walking school bus.

WALKABLE-COMMUNITY INFORMATION

America WALKS, Portland, Oregon. This nonprofit coalition promotes the benefits of walking and the development of local and regional pedestrian advocacy groups. Call 503-222-1077 or visit www.americawalks.org.

Pedestrian and Bicycle Information Center, Washington, D.C. Information on creating facilities and environments for more walking and bicycling and improving safety for pedestrians and cyclists. Web site includes an online neighborhood walkability checklist. Call 202-463-8405 or visit www.walkinginfo.org.

The Rails-to-Trails Conservancy, Washington, D.C. A national advocacy organization working to convert abandoned rail beds into multi-use trails, the RTC has facilitated the creation of more than 15,000 miles of rail-trails nationwide. Call 800-888-7747 or visit www.railtrails.org.

Walkable Communities, Inc., High Springs, Florida. A consulting firm run by Dan Burden—one of the nation's walkable-community experts—that can help your community envision and implement a more livable future. Call 904-454-3304 or visit www.walkable.org.

WATER (HYDRATION SYSTEMS)

Aquifer vest by Ultimate Direction. 800-426-7229; www.ultimatedirection.com

Camelbak. Back and waist-worn packs by Camelbak. 800-767-8725; www.camelbak.com/rec/f_rec_search.htm

Index